Concepts of
Mental Disorder

A Continuing Debate

The contributions in this book derive from papers given at a symposium, "Concepts of Mental Disorder", October 1989, augmented by chapters by Drs Tyrer and Snaith. The book has been sponsored by the Mental Health Unit, Newcastle upon Tyne, United Kingdom, and particular thanks are due to its Chief Executive, Mr Lionel Joyce, for his help and support. Technical assistance given by Ralph Footring, Scientific Editor, Royal College of Psychiatrists, is gratefully acknowledged.

Edited by
ALAN KERR
HAMISH McCLELLAND

Concepts of Mental Disorder

A Continuing Debate

GASKELL

©The Royal College of Psychiatrists 1991

ISBN 0 902241 38 9

Gaskell is an imprint of the Royal College of Psychiatrists,
17 Belgrave Square, London SW1

Distributed in North America
by American Psychiatric Press, Inc.
ISBN 0 88048 605 8

British Library Cataloguing in Publication Data
Concepts of mental disorder.
1. Humans. Mental disorders
I. Kerr, Alan   II. McClelland, Hamish   III. Royal College
of Psychiatrists
616.89

ISBN 0-902241-38-9

Phototypeset by Dobbie Typesetting Limited, Tavistock, Devon
Printed in Great Britain

Contents

Contributors

Timothy J. Crow, Head of Division of Psychiatry, Clinical Research Centre, Watford Road, Harrow, Middlesex

Steven R. Hirsch, Professor, Department of Psychiatry, Charing Cross and Westminster Medical School, St Dunstan's Road, London

David Kay, Emeritus Professor of Psychiatry, MRC Neurochemical Pathology Unit, Newcastle General Hospital, Newcastle upon Tyne

Robert E. Kendell, Professor, University Department of Psychiatry, The Kennedy Tower, Royal Edinburgh Hospital, Morningside Park, Edinburgh

Alan Kerr, Consultant Psychiatrist, St Nicholas Hospital, Gosforth, Newcastle upon Tyne

Gerald L. Klerman, Professor of Psychiatry, Associate Chairman for Research, Cornell University Medical College, The New York Hospital, Payne Whitney Clinic, 525 East 68th Street, New York, USA

Hamish McClelland, Consultant Psychiatrist, St Nicholas Hospital, Gosforth, Newcastle upon Tyne

Robin M. Murray, Professor, Department of Psychological Medicine, Institute of Psychiatry, De Crespigny Park, London

Eadbhard O'Callaghan, Research Psychiatrist, Institute of Psychiatry, De Crespigny Park, London

Kenneth Rawnsley, CBE, Emeritus Professor of Psychological Medicine, University of Wales College of Medicine, Cardiff

Sir Martin Roth, Emeritus Professor, Department of Psychiatry, University of Cambridge, Addenbrooke's Hospital, Level 5, Hills Road, Cambridge

Philip Snaith, Senior Lecturer, Department of Psychiatry, St James's University Hospital, Leeds

Erik Strömgren, Professor, Institute of Psychiatric Demography, Psychiatric Hospital, 8240 Risskov, Denmark

Peter Tyrer, Consultant Psychiatrist, St Charles's Hospital, London

Myrna M. Weissman, Professor, College of Physicians and Surgeons of Columbia University, 722 West 168th Street, Box 14, New York, USA

Foreword

KENNETH RAWNSLEY

It was my privilege to chair the meeting organised by the Mental Health Unit of Newcastle Health Authority and held in Newcastle upon Tyne in October 1989 from which most of the chapters in this book were derived.

The main topic was the status of schizophrenia and of affective illness within the field of psychotic disorders. Are they distinct disease entities, or points on a continuum of psychotic morbidity, or what? Is schizophrenia a single condition or does the term subsume a variety of ailments? And where do the reactive psychoses important in Scandinavian psychiatry fit into the rubrics? The limits of affective disorder are also a matter for debate. Severe depression with delusions, hypomania, the 'minor' depressions and anxiety disorders which form the bread and butter of psychiatric morbidity in general practice: are they all variants of a single disorder?

I listened to the arguments, advanced with great skill and sometimes with a degree of passion, from all conceivable angles. An early edition of the programme for the Newcastle meeting labelled my final contribution from the chair as "Adjudication". Mercifully this was later amended to "Comments and closing remarks". My secret judgement would have been the Scottish verdict of "Not proven". Yet, at the end of the day, my mood was one of cautious optimism. I detected a fruitful tension between the realists and the nominalists and a willingness to pursue their quest using the full armamentarium of epidemiology, genetics, psychopathology and brain studies.

Introduction

ALAN KERR and HAMISH McCLELLAND

Disputes about concepts and appropriate models of mental disorders extend back to classical time. The nature of the differing approaches of the two main philosophical schools has altered little and remains clearly evident to this day: that which led to a view of medical disorders as disease entities (the Platonic tradition), and that emphasising the natural history in individual patients (the Hippocratic (Aristotelian) tradition). The latter, continuum view of mental disorder holds that the differences found relate to variations in chronicity and severity, while the former, categorical approach holds that there are distinct disease entities and that valid and useful lines of demarcation can be drawn between them. A third viewpoint would be to acknowledge the presence of dimensional and categorical components in a single framework.

Nevertheless, all such viewpoints implicitly accept the need to classify. Unless we recognise similarities by groupings the world loses meaning as each object remains unique. In the scientific world, classification is necessary for economy of memory, ease of manipulation of objects, and the generation of hypotheses (Jablensky, 1988). When a classification system grows out of, and is applied to, biological disorders it must both be rigorously scientific and be of value to the practising physician.

On the other hand, classifications based on consensus will fail because they are contaminated by compromise and likely self-contradiction (e.g. the World Health Organization's *International Classification of Diseases*) and classifications that are too practical fail to be heuristic. An example of the latter is given in the chapter by Peter Tyrer of his senior, who classified mental disorders according to their response to treatment. Classification is pragmatic and poses no conceptual problems where, as in overt organic disorders, the causation by underlying pathology is clear. However, where aetiology cannot be demonstrated in tangible form, there is scope for disagreement between the traditional views. The central area of controversy has been in the area of the psychoses and related disorders. Repeated attempts to resolve disputes have been made on the basis of detailed clinical and outcome studies. In recent years such data have been subjected to sophisticated statistical techniques such as discriminant function analysis, but without resolution of the differences.

In the present volume the contributors reflect widely differing viewpoints in a debate that has its origins in the beginning of modern psychiatry, in the middle of the 19th century. While clinical and prognostic studies remain important in trying to resolve these issues, increasing attention has been given of late to more independent lines of inquiry, such as genetic and neuropathological studies. However, the interpretation of these data has varied, as have views on the appropriate lines of demarcation within the psychoses, and whether the traditional boundaries between schizophrenia, schizoaffective disorder and affective psychoses should be maintained. Of special interest have been recent observations from neuropathological studies in support of an organic basis for Kraepelin's original concept of dementia praecox (Roberts, 1991). Partly under the influence of Kraepelin and Schneider, who excluded the neuroses and personality disorders from the realm of mental illness, these conditions have received less conceptual scrutiny than the psychoses. But similar disagreements are apparent there also.

Here we have aimed to provide a forum for debate of views on how mental disorders should be conceptualised. The first two chapters address the heart of the debate, with Professor Kendell elucidating the continuum (nominalist) viewpoint and Professor Sir Martin Roth arguing for the realist view and emphasising how this approach enables the validity of the concepts to be tested. Between them they also sketch the historical and philosophical dimensions to these questions. Dr Crow then takes up the continuum hypothesis, setting it out from a genetic basis and advancing his own hypothesis; Professor Murray and Dr O'Callaghan also examine the genetic evidence, along with the neuropathological findings, and propose that separate entities be accepted, but in doing so redraw the conventional boundaries. Professor Hirsch recommends, however, that the focus should be on syndromes, rather than on diagnostic groups, and on investigation of the underlying disturbances of function and subsets of clinical phenomena. The arguments are then looked at from different perspectives by Professors Klerman and Strömgren. Professor Klerman describes the profound change of thinking in the United States since World War II which has led to the current ascendancy of the neo-Kraepelinian approach and the introduction of DSM–III by the American Psychiatric Association. Professor Strömgren traces German thinking since the emergence of the concept of *Einheitspsychose* (unitary psychosis) 150 years ago, and makes a special plea for the retention of the Scandinavian concept of the reactive psychoses. Professor Kay reviews the contribution that studies of psychosis in old age have made to this debate in terms of a lifetime longitudinal perspective and also genetic evidence. Professor Weissman proposes that a categorical distinction be made within the affective psychoses on the basis of data on heredity. Finally, Dr Tyrer puts forward a unitary view of the neuroses and personality disorders, based on clinical, outcome, treatment, and genetic information, and Dr Snaith places the current classification of these conditions in a historical context.

Our contributors illustrate in their diversity of views the uncertain but exciting state of current psychiatric classification. Such diversity does not come from minds wildly extrapolating beyond the limits of contemporary knowledge. If there is one message from this volume it is that psychiatry is in ferment. A flood of information from advances in genetics, neuropathology, non-invasive investigatory techniques and epidemiology has not yet been properly integrated and so has overwhelmed our ability to conceptualise and organise the data.

''For the advancement of medical science the delineation of syndromes without prior commitment to views on causation, is a well tried starting point for studies to elucidate pathogenesis and aetiology, and extend the area within which practice can be based on objective biological knowledge'' (Scadding, 1990). A major step in the clarification of thinking about psychiatric classification was the separation of syndrome from aetiology (Essen-Möller & Wohlfahrt, 1947) and this differentiation is accommodated within the contemporary multi-axial approach to classification. With the impending implementation of ICD–10 and DSM–IV, thinking about the theoretical models and concepts implicit in these systems seems especially relevant at this time.

Will the next decade deflate our optimism that we are near to major breakthrough in our understanding of mental disorder? If a breakthrough does come, will it be through patient trial and error, or will there be some sudden, creative leap that is immediately accepted by researchers and clinicians alike? If and when a paradigm shift arises, will it be based on evidence that is around us now, so that we, like Huxley on closing his copy of the *Origin of Species*, will exclaim ''How extremely stupid of me not to have thought of that''?

References

ESSEN-MÖLLER, E. & WOHLFAHRT, S. (1947) Suggestions for the amendment of the official Swedish classification of mental disorders. *Eighth Congress of Scandinavian Psychiatrists*, **47**, 551–555.

JABLENSKY, A. (1988) Methodological issues in psychiatric classification. *British Journal of Psychiatry*, **152** (suppl. 1), 15–20.

ROBERTS, G. W. (1991) Schizophrenia: a neuropathological perspective. *British Journal of Psychiatry*, **158**, 8–17.

SCADDING, J. G. (1990) The semantic problems of psychiatry. *Psychological Medicine*, **20**, 243–248.

1 The major functional psychoses: are they independent entities or part of a continuum? Philosophical and conceptual issues underlying the debate

ROBERT E. KENDELL

The relationship between the functional psychoses is not often discussed, and discussion of that relationship raises fundamental issues that are rarely considered or debated by psychiatrists. In particular, it involves the usually unwitting assumptions made about the nature of mental illness, and of disease in general.

Historical origins

Schizophrenia and manic–depressive or affective psychosis are fundamentally Kraepelin's concepts. He and most of his contemporaries took it for granted that the variegated and shifting forms of mental illness with which they were confronted, or at least the various forms of insanity with which they were primarily concerned, consisted of a finite number of 'disease entities', each with a distinct pattern of symptoms and course, and with distinct causes, treatments and neuropathologies waiting to be discovered. Even in his own generation, however, there were a few discordant voices questioning these assumptions. August Hoche, for example, made this tart commentary on Kraepelin's classification and the enthusiastic reception it was then receiving:

> "A kind of thought compulsion, a logical and aesthetic necessity, insists that we seek for well-defined, self-contained disease entities, but here as elsewhere, unfortunately, our subjective need is no proof of the reality of that which we desire, no proof that these pure types do, in point of fact actually occur." (Hoche, 1910)

In his mature years, even Kraepelin himself began to have doubts about the validity of the distinction he had drawn between dementia praecox and manic–depressive insanity. Referring to "the difficulties which still prevent us from distinguishing reliably between manic depressive insanity and dementia praecox" he observed that:

1

> "no experienced psychiatrist will deny that there is an alarmingly large number of cases in which it seems impossible, in spite of the most careful observation, to make a firm diagnosis . . . it is becoming increasingly clear that we cannot distinguish satisfactorily between these two illnesses and this brings home the suspicion that our formulation of the problem may be incorrect." (Kraepelin, 1920)

These doubts were immediately followed, however, by a firm insistence that "we must at all costs adhere to the basic difference between the disease processes concerned". Kraepelin clearly realised, as many others have subsequently done, that dementia praecox and manic–depressive illness were the twin pillars on which the whole of his classification depended, and that anyone who disturbed those pillars was in danger of bringing the whole edifice crashing down around him.

Realists and nominalists

It is important to appreciate that this dispute between Kraepelin and Hoche was simply one manifestation of a much broader conflict between two ancient philosophical traditions, variously known as Platonic and Aristotelian, realist and nominalist, rationalist and empirical. In medicine this dispute has been focused on the concept of 'disease entities'. Realists maintain that such things exist and are usually bent on identifying them; nominalists regard them as man-made abstractions, justified only by their convenience and sometimes a dangerous source of misconceptions.

In medicine the 17th-century English physician Thomas Sydenham was the supreme realist. Kahlbaum and Kraepelin and their contemporaries were simply following in his footsteps. It was Sydenham who first insisted that diseases "were to be reduced to certain and determinate kinds with the same exactness as we see it done by botanic writers in their treatises of plants", and that this could be done by virtue of "certain distinguishing signs which nature has particularly fixed to every species". The nominalist stance, on the other hand, was epitomised by Rousseau's remark a century later that "Il n'y a pas de maladie, il n'y a que des malades" – there are no illnesses, only sick people.

These two schools of thought have always been in conflict, partly because they have rarely understood one another. As Karl Jaspers (1959) observed:

> "the battle between the two camps has been fought with a good deal of mutual contempt and everyone was convinced of the total fiasco created by the endeavours of the opposite camp. Yet in view of the actual history we may suspect . . . that both camps were on the track of something valid and could well complement each other instead of wrangling."

Jaspers went on to raise the issue of whether there are only stages and variants of a single *Einheitspsychose* (unitary psychosis) or a series of disease entities – and came to a very interesting conclusion whose relevance has not lessened with the passage of time:

> "There are neither. The latter view is right in so far that the idea of disease entities has become a fruitful orientation for the investigations of special psychiatry. The former view is right in so far that no actual disease entities exist in scientific psychiatry."

This characteristically perceptive remark goes some way to explain why the debate continues and the issue remains unresolved.

The nominalist position

I must now sketch out my own, nominalist, viewpoint, and start by insisting that the question underlying much of the debate in this book, "Are the major functional psychoses independent or are they part of a continuum?", is both misleading and meaningless, and could only have been framed by a realist. First, and most basically, we are not discussing the fundamental nature of the phenomena we call 'mental illness'. We are merely discussing the 'models' we construct, or invent, as convenient representations of those phenomena. 'Schizophrenia' and 'manic–depressive illness', and all our other diagnostic terms, are simply concepts. They are products of human imagination and they exist only in the realm of ideas. The only fundamental question we can ask about them, therefore, is whether they are useful concepts, and even that question has to be qualified further – useful to whom, and in what context?

Secondly, the question – "Are the major functional psychoses independent or part of a continuum?" – is a confusing condensation of what ought to be two quite distinct questions. All classifications of mental disorders are fundamentally 'models' which we use to represent the variation in symptoms, in course, and in response to treatment which we observe in our patients. In choosing which model or classification to use, the first decision we have to make is whether to use a typology (a set of categories) or a dimensional model (a set of continua). If we choose a typology we then have to decide how many categories we wish to distinguish. A typology of functional psychoses might, for example, consist of only one category – the *Einheitspsychose* of Zeller and Griesinger (see Chapters 2 and 7). Alternatively, it might consist of two categories – Kraepelin's dementia praecox and manic–depressive insanity. Or it might consist of three or more categories; we might decide to add Leonhard's cycloid psychoses, or a group of reactive psychoses, to Kraepelin's two major groupings. Similarly, if we choose a dimensional model we must decide how many dimensions we wish to recognise, and whether or not these are to be orthogonal. But whichever model we choose, none is right or wrong. Different models are likely, however, to vary considerably in their usefulness, depending on how well the properties of the model match the phenomena we observe in our patients, and on whether the empirical questions they prompt us to ask prove to be fertile or sterile.

Throughout this century the most widely used classification, or model, of mental illness has been a typology with at least two categories of functional psychosis, which we have called schizophrenia and manic–depressive (affective) psychosis. Some psychiatrists – the realists – have assumed, like Kraepelin, that these were two distinct disease entities. Others – the nominalists – have regarded them simply as concepts which helped us to think coherently about the varied phenomena of psychosis, and to communicate with one another.

But even if we adopt the nominalist position, as most contemporary scientists and philosophers now do, it is still an important question whether the discontinuity in the model – the distinction between schizophrenia and affective illness – corresponds to a discontinuity in the observable phenomena of illness. We want to know, in other words, whether we are carving nature at one of its joints. If we are, our classification is likely to help us to understand and to predict; if we are not, it is likely to mislead us. This, I suggest, is the central question.

The search for a 'point of rarity'

At present, both schizophrenia and affective psychosis are purely clinical concepts, in the sense that both continue to be defined by their symptoms – a mixture of observable abnormalities of behaviour and descriptions of abnormal or distressing subjective experiences. The question of whether or not there is a natural boundary between these two psychoses therefore resolves itself into the empirical question of whether patients with a mixture of the symptoms of schizophrenic and affective psychoses are more or less common than those who possess only the symptoms of one or the other. In brief, the issue is whether the 'greys' are more or less frequent than the 'blacks' and the 'whites'. In graphical terms the question is whether, when variation in symptom patterns is reduced to a single linear dimension, the distribution of patients on that dimension is unimodal, or bimodal (with a 'point of rarity' in the middle).

The most convenient statistical technique for maximising the likelihood of generating a bimodal distribution of scores on a linear dimension is discriminant function analysis (Rao, 1948) and in the 1970s I and my colleagues at the Institute of Psychiatry tried with several different data sets to obtain a bimodal distribution, but without success. Our first attempt

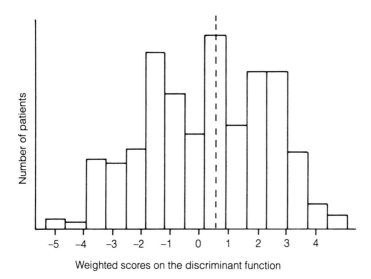

Fig. 1.1. Scores of 146 schizophrenics and 146 manic–depressives (unipolar and bipolar) on a discriminant function derived from those 292 patients (from Kendell & Gourlay, 1970). The trimodal distribution cannot be interpreted as evidence for the presence of a third population – if patients with some unidentified third disorder had been present, there is no reason why their scores should cluster at any particular point on the function

was based on the ratings on the Present State Examination of 292 subjects studied by the US/UK Diagnostic Project (Kendell & Gourlay, 1970). They were actually all patients with a project team diagnosis of schizophrenia or affective psychosis in two consecutive series each of 146 hospital admissions, one to a London mental hospital and the other to a New York state hospital. The overall distribution of scores on the discriminant function differed significantly from a normal distribution, but it was trimodal rather than bimodal (Fig. 1.1).

Our second attempt a few years later was based on the English patients from the original combined New York and London series (Brockington *et al*, 1979). As these patients had been followed up and reinterviewed six to seven years after their index admission, ratings of course and outcome were available on 128 patients, in addition to ratings of symptoms. Probably because of the inclusion of these course and outcome ratings, a bimodal distribution of scores was obtained on the discriminant function this time (Fig. 1.2).

By itself, however, this proves nothing. Because the separation obtained between any two populations is spuriously increased by what are in fact chance differences between them, the analysis always has to be cross-validated by applying the item weights of the discriminant function to a second population of patients who have not contributed to the derivation

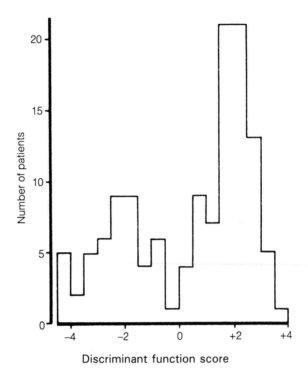

Fig. 1.2. Scores of 128 patients with functional psychoses on a discriminant function derived from the 36 patients in that series with outcome diagnoses of schizophrenia and the 43 with outcome diagnoses of affective psychosis (from Brockington et al, 1979)

of these weights. When this was done with a series of 106 patients with schizoaffective illnesses the distribution was skewed but unimodal (Fig. 1.3).

When a second discriminant function was derived from these 106 schizoaffective patients the distribution of their scores on that function was ambiguous. To casual inspection it was skewed but unimodal; however, statistical modelling showed that the observed distribution of scores could be accounted for better by two overlapping populations than by one. The same happened when this second discriminant function (derived from the 106 schizoaffective patients) was cross-validated on the original 128 schizophrenic and affective patients. The distribution again appeared skewed but unimodal; and again statistical modelling suggested that the observed distribution could be better accounted for by two overlapping distributions than by one (Fig. 1.4).

Although this series of discriminant function analyses failed to generate an unequivocally bimodal distribution of scores at any stage, it is important to appreciate that this does not prove that schizophrenic and affective psychoses are not distinct disorders. Discriminant function analysis can

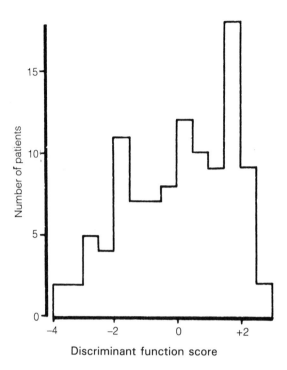

Fig. 1.3. Scores of 106 patients with schizoaffective illnesses on a discriminant function derived previously from criterion groups with outcome diagnoses of schizophrenia (n = 36) and affective psychosis (n = 43) (from Brockington et al, *1979)*

never do this, because it is always possible that a different selection of discriminatory items would generate a bimodal distribution.

In fact Cloninger *et al* (1985) in St Louis have succeeded in generating a bimodal distribution of scores, using ratings derived from no less than 1749 subjects – a consecutive series of 500 psychiatric out-patients and 1249 of their first-degree relatives. Using data from half these subjects they generated a discriminant function to distinguish schizophrenia from a combination of all other mental disorders and the absence of any disorder, rather than to distinguish schizophrenic from affective psychoses as I and my colleagues had always done. Their bimodal distribution held up on cross-validation or replication with the other 50% of their subjects and they also obtained a bimodal distribution when they plotted the scores of the subgroup of subjects with schizophrenic or affective psychoses (Fig. 1.5).

The St Louis group has therefore presented good evidence that schizophrenia is a discrete disorder, separated from other conditions by a natural boundary or 'point of rarity'. However, their original symptom ratings were derived from semistructured interviews which may not have

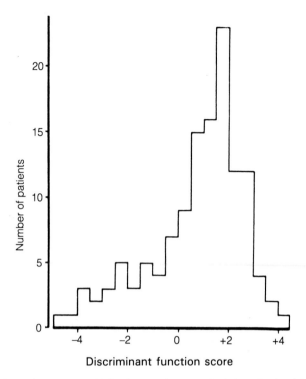

Fig. 1.4. Scores of 128 patients with functional psychoses on a discriminant function derived previously from schizoaffectives with agreed 'forced-choice' outcome diagnoses of schizophrenia (n = 35) and affective psychosis (n = 47) (from Brockington et al, 1979)

prevented them being biased by the diagnostic preconceptions of the clinicians involved; and no other research group has yet repeated the demonstration. So there must still be some doubt whether the matter is finally proven.

Relationship between syndrome and aetiology

Although both schizophrenic and affective psychoses are currently defined by their clinical syndromes, we are intensely interested in their underlying aetiology, and look forward to the time when both conditions will be defined at some more fundamental level; by their neuropathology perhaps, or by some characteristic genetic or neurophysiological abnormality. Our arguments about the relationship between the two syndromes are therefore always likely to be coloured by our assumptions about the relationships between their aetiologies. Psychiatrists, like Professor Sir Martin Roth (Chapter 2), who maintain that schizophrenia and manic–depressive psychosis are distinct

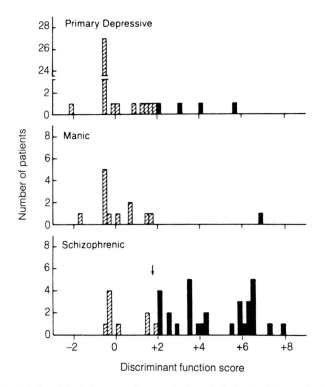

Fig. 1.5. *Distribution of discriminant scores in schizophrenics and affective disorder in a replication sample:* ■ *subjects with scores in the schizophrenic range (greater than* + 2) *regardless of actual diagnosis;* ▨ *patients with scores in the non-schizophrenic range, again regardless of actual diagnosis. The arrow indicates the point of rarity (from Cloninger* et al *(1985),* ©*1985, American Medical Association)*

entities are, I suspect, not really making statements about symptom clusters. They are proclaiming their belief that the two syndromes will eventually be shown to have quite distinct aetiologies. It is certainly true that disorders with quite different aetiologies may have identical, or indistinguishable, syndromes. Retinitis pigmentosa is an obvious example. In fact, the relationship between symptoms and aetiology is inconstant and unpredictable, and inferences from the one to the other, in either direction, may prove incorrect. We know that Huntington's chorea is transmitted by a single dominant gene with virtually complete penetrance, yet the psychiatric disorders associated with it are very diverse, ranging from schizophrenia to major depression, dysthymia, and personality disorders of various kinds (Caine & Shoulson, 1983). A single genotype may thus be associated with a variety of psychiatric syndromes. Although concordance is much commoner than discordance, there are a number of well documented examples of pairs of monozygous twins with different psychiatric disorders. There is also evidence that the dominant autosomal gene responsible for Tourette's syndrome may manifest itself as obsessive–compulsive disorder as well as, or even instead of, Tourette's syndrome itself or other motor tics (Pauls *et al*, 1986).

Despite these sobering examples, much of our research is basically an attempt to identify stable relationships between clinical syndromes and other variables. Sometimes we are only interested in predicting outcome or response to treatment. But often we are searching for clues to aetiology and this search has often resulted in unwarranted conclusions. Many investigators, having found that samples of patients with two different syndromes, X and Y, differed significantly on some other variable like age at onset, or prognosis, or ventricular brain ratio, or response to dexamethasone, have argued that this is evidence that X and Y are distinct entities. The conclusion does not follow, any more than a demonstration that samples of clever men and of stupid men differed significantly in height, or average salary or mean age at death, or all three, would constitute evidence that clever men and stupid men belonged to different species. Strictly speaking, all that has been demonstrated in either case is that the two are not both random samples from the same population. Before we are entitled to conclude that there is something fundamentally different between syndromes X and Y we have to show that the relationship between symptoms and age at onset, or prognosis, or ventricular brain ratio, or response to dexamethasone, is non-linear.

Significance of non-linear relationships

Brockington and I have tried to demonstrate a non-linear relationship between the outcome of the functional psychoses and their symptoms (Kendell & Brockington, 1980). As before, we used scores on a discriminant function as a convenient means of converting the variation in symptoms between schizophrenic and affective psychoses to a linear variable. We then divided an unselected series of 127 patients with functional psychoses for whom we had extensive follow-up data into ten subgroups occupying different loci along this dimension and calculated the mean scores of each of these ten subgroups on six different measures of outcome. On all six measures outcome was worse at the schizophrenic than at the affective end of the scale, but on none of the six was there a convincing discontinuity in the relationship between outcome and symptoms (Fig. 1.6). If only because the variance in outcome was so high on most of the indices, the gradient in outcome was compatible with a linear relationship for all six (Fig. 1.7).

As with failure to demonstrate bimodality in symptoms, this does not prove that schizophrenic and affective psychoses are not distinct conditions. For one thing, it is always possible that a non-linear relationship could be demonstrated using some other criterion variable, one derived from sensory-evoked potentials, perhaps, or the proportion of patients in whom a particular genetic abnormality was identified.

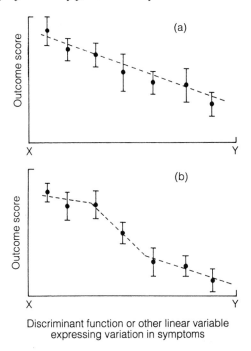

Fig. 1.6. (a) Linear and (b) non-linear relationships between outcome (or some alternative criterion variable) and symptoms (from Kendell & Brockington, 1980)

A family study by Tsuang *et al* (1980) in Iowa serves to illustrate the fallacy I am concerned with. Tsuang and his colleagues located and interviewed 1578 first-degree relatives of 200 schizophrenics, 100 manics and 225 depressives who had all been admitted to psychiatric hospitals in Iowa between 1934 and 1944. They also interviewed the relatives of 160 surgical controls admitted to hospital for appendicectomy or herniorrhaphy in the same decade. They found an increased morbid risk of schizophrenia, but not of affective illness, in the first-degree relatives of their schizophrenic probands, and an increased morbid risk of affective illness, but not of schizophrenia, in the relatives of their affective probands. In many ways the study design was exemplary, and a considerable advance on previous family studies. The diagnoses of the probands were based on operational criteria (similar to the Feighner criteria), the relatives were interviewed blind to proband diagnosis, and the numbers involved were substantial. For this reason Tsuang's evidence that both schizophrenic and affective disorders 'breed true' has often been cited as compelling evidence that they are distinct disorders. However, the original 525 psychiatric probands were picked from a much larger population of 3800 consecutive admissions. They were the patients with textbook illnesses, and those with schizoaffective symptoms and atypical illnesses of other kinds were omitted. Only if Tsuang had included

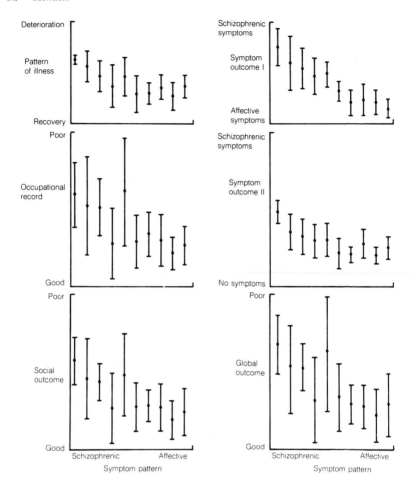

Fig. 1.7. Relationship between symptoms and outcome in 127 patients with functional psychoses using six different indices of outcome (from Kendell & Brockington, 1980)

probands across the whole range of psychotic symptoms, assigned them to a series of loci along a schizoaffective continuum, and then demonstrated a discontinuity in the relatives' morbid risk at some point on that continuum, would he and we have been entitled to conclude that schizophrenic and affective psychoses had been shown to be genetically distinct disorders.

Conclusions

I have tried to describe some of the philosophical and conceptual issues raised by the debate surrounding our concepts of mental disorder, and to clarify the kinds of evidence needed to establish the presence of a valid boundary between two related syndromes like schizophrenic and affective psychoses. I have also underlined my own nominalist viewpoint. If schizophrenic and affective psychoses do eventually prove to have distinct aetiologies I will rejoice, for many intractable problems will thereby be solved, or simply become irrelevant. At present, however, we have no compelling reason to believe that they are distinct in either their symptom patterns or their aetiology. For the last 20 years I have been dismayed by the widespread assumption that schizophrenia and manic–depressive illness are distinct diseases simply because we have given them different names, because the distinction between them is regarded as an important matter in everyday clinical practice, and because they are usually treated differently. I have therefore tried again and again to convince my students and colleagues that these assumptions are unjustified and that we must be prepared to consider other possibilities, and to think in dimensional terms.

As a consequence of the uncritical acceptance of the Kraepelinian dichotomy, interest has generally been focused on the differences between the two syndromes, and how to distinguish them, rather than on their similarities. In fact, these similarities are rather impressive. Schizophrenic and manic–depressive (bipolar) disorders have similar ages of onset. Both characteristically develop in late adolescence or early adult life, yet both may develop at any time up to late middle age. Because 'interforms' between the two – Schneider's *Zwischenfalle* or our schizoaffective disorders – are so common, we have great difficulty deciding where to draw the boundary between them, and in practice successive generations of psychiatrists have moved that boundary first one way and then the other. Moreover, each syndrome may be transformed into the other by the passage of time. Patients who originally present with the typical symptoms of schizophrenia may subsequently pursue a characteristically affective course, and vice versa (Sheldrick *et al*, 1977). And although the lifetime prognosis of schizophrenic disorders is, on average, consistently worse than that of affective psychoses, the prognoses of the two have, nonetheless, much in common. Both are usually lifelong illnesses and the typical course of each consists of a series of psychotic episodes occurring at unpredictable intervals throughout adult life. Yet single episodes without any recurrence are well documented for both. Major genetic factors are involved in the aetiology of both syndromes, yet at the same time life events have been shown in both to play a role in the precipitation of individual episodes. Although both disorders tend to run in families, neither 'breeds true' (Stassen *et al*, 1988): each contaminates the other. There are also well documented examples of pairs of monozygotic twins, one of whom had a schizophrenic illness while the other's symptoms were consistently affective (McGuffin *et al*, 1987).

The difference in the response of the two syndromes to therapeutic agents is also much less impressive than our treatment conventions would suggest.

The double-blind trials that have been conducted in the last decade have shown that the therapeutic effects of electroconvulsive therapy (ECT) are indistinguishable in severe depression, mania and acute schizophrenia. In all three syndromes the therapeutic effect is genuine, and sometimes dramatic, but also relatively short-lived. Both in schizophrenia and in depression the difference between real and simulated ECT is undetectable after three or four months (Brandon *et al*, 1984; Abraham & Kulhara, 1987). Because neuroleptics are usually reserved for schizophrenic illnesses and lithium and antidepressants for affective illnesses comparatively little is known about the effect of these drugs on the other syndrome. Yet some of the early trials of the phenothiazines and tricyclic antidepressants suggested that the symptoms of both schizophrenic and depressive illnesses could be alleviated by both imipramine and chlorpromazine or thioridazine (Klein & Fink, 1963; Overall *et al*, 1964). The Northwick Park functional psychosis trial also demonstrated that pimozide was equally effective in relieving delusions and hallucinations whether these were in the setting of a schizophrenic or an affective psychosis, while lithium relieved elevation of mood equally well in both mania and schizophrenia (Johnstone *et al*, 1988).

It is sometimes said that the most accurate measure of a scientist's stature is the length of time after his death that his reputation inhibits further progress in his discipline. The aphorism is as true of psychiatry as it is of physics. In their different ways the towering reputations of both Freud and Kraepelin have discouraged intelligent appraisal of the phenomena of mental illness, by inhibiting us from worrying about things which were incompatible with their teaching. But, as Kuhn observed, progress in science – the development of new paradigms – is usually crucially dependent on new explanatory hypotheses for those inconvenient facts not accounted for by the prevailing paradigm.

I suggest, therefore, that it is time we questioned Kraepelin's paradigm of distinct disease entities and of two discrete types of functional psychosis. The concepts of schizophrenia and manic–depressive psychosis have undoubtedly been useful to several generations of clinicians and it is still possible that Kraepelin's fundamental assumptions about the psychoses will be vindicated. On the other hand, the stultifying effects of these assumptions are increasingly apparent. For most of this century they have resulted in patients whose symptoms did not fit either of his rubrics being forced into one of two alternative Procrustean beds. They have led to the development of therapeutic conventions which are not justified by the results of clinical trials, and to inappropriate aetiological assumptions, like the dopamine theory of schizophrenia, derived from these conventions. They have also repeatedly led to inappropriate research strategies. Time after time research workers have compared groups of schizophrenics and normal controls and found some difference between the two which they assumed to be a clue to the aetiology of schizophrenia, only for someone else, years later, to find the same abnormality in patients with affective psychoses. Of all the dozens of biological abnormalities reported in schizophrenics in the last 50 years, none has yet proved to be specific to that syndrome. All have been found, although often less frequently, in patients with affective psychoses, and none has been demonstrated in more than a minority of schizophrenics.

The evidence to support Kraepelin's *Zweiteilungsprinzip* is too flimsy to justify putting all our eggs in that one basket. To maximise our chances of elucidating the aetiology of the psychoses we must be prepared to entertain, and to experiment with, alternative ways of classifying psychotic illnesses. The continuum model is based on a wealth of empirical evidence that the numerous patients whose symptoms are intermediate between those of the classic schizophrenic and affective stereotypes are also intermediate in treatment response, in long-term outcome, and in the pattern of illness found in their first-degree relatives. The particular version of the model which Dr Crow persuasively advocates in Chapter 3 has the great virtue of generating predictions which are precise and testable, and is therefore readily falsifiable. It also forces us to envisage alternatives to the familiar dichotomy which we have taken for granted for too long. For that reason alone it is most welcome.

At the end of the day I would be happy for today's realists, Roth, Winokur and Kendler, to be proved correct, just as Sydenham was correct in maintaining that measles and scarlet fever were distinct conditions. But at present I do not consider that their assumptions and convictions are justified by the evidence available to us.

References

ABRAHAM, K. R. & KULHARA, P. (1987) The efficacy of electroconvulsive therapy in the treatment of schizophrenia: a comparative study. *British Journal of Psychiatry*, **151**, 152–155.

BRANDON, S., COWLEY, P., McDONALD, C., *et al* (1984) Electroconvulsive therapy: results in depressive illness from the Leicestershire trial. *British Medical Journal*, **288**, 22–25.

BROCKINGTON, I. F., KENDELL, R. E., WAINWRIGHT, S., *et al* (1979) The distinction between the affective psychoses and schizophrenia. *British Journal of Psychiatry*, **135**, 243–248.

CAINE, E. D. & SHOULSON, I. (1983) Psychiatric syndromes in Huntington's disease. *American Journal of Psychiatry*, **140**, 728–733.

CLONINGER, C. R., MARTIN, R. L., GUZE, S. B., *et al* (1985) Diagnosis and prognosis in schizophrenia. *Archives of General Psychiatry*, **42**, 15–25.

HOCHE, A. (1910) Die Melancholiefrage. *Zentralblatt für Nervenheilkunde*, **21**, 193–203.

JASPERS, K. (1959) *Allgemeine Psychopathologie* (7th edn) (trans. (1962) J. Hoenig & M. W. Hamilton. Manchester: Manchester University Press).

JOHNSTONE, E. C., CROW, T. J., FRITH, C. D., *et al* (1988) The Northwick Park 'functional' psychosis study: diagnosis and treatment response. *Lancet*, **ii**, 119–124.

KENDELL, R. E. & GOURLAY, J. (1970) The clinical distinction between the affective psychoses and schizophrenia. *British Journal of Psychiatry*, **117**, 261–266.

—— & BROCKINGTON, I. F. (1980) The identification of disease entities and the relationship between schizophrenic and affective psychoses. *British Journal of Psychiatry*, **137**, 324–331.

KLEIN, D. F. & FINK, M. (1963) Multiple item factors as change measures in psychopharmacology. *Psychopharmacologia*, **4**, 43–52.

KRAEPELIN, E. (1920) Die Erscheinungsformen des Irreseins. *Zeitschrift für die gesamte Neurologie und Psychiatrie*, **62**, 1–29. (English trans. (1974) in *Themes and Variations in European Psychiatry* (eds S. R. Hirsch & M. Shepherd). Bristol: John Wright.)

MCGUFFIN, P., MURRAY, R. M. & REVELEY, A. M. (1987) Genetic influence on the psychoses. In *Recurrent and Chronic Psychoses* (ed. T. J. Crow). *British Medical Bulletin*, **43**, 531–556.

OVERALL, J. E., HOLLISTER, L. E., MEYER, F., *et al* (1964) Imipramine and thioridazine in depressed and schizophrenic patients. *Journal of the American Medical Association*, **189**, 605–608.

PAULS, D. L., TOWBIN, K. E., LECKMAN, J. F., *et al* (1986) Gilles de la Tourette's syndrome and obscure compulsive disorder: evidence supporting a genetic relationship. *Archives of General Psychiatry*, **43**, 1180–1182.

RAO, C. R. (1948) The utilisation of multiple measurements in problems of biological classification. *Journal of the Royal Statistical Society*, B, **10**, 159–193.

SHELDRICK, C., JABLENSKY, A., SARTORIUS, N., *et al* (1977) Schizophrenia succeeded by affective illness: catamnestic study and statistical enquiry. *Psychological Medicine*, **7**, 619–624.

STASSEN, H. H., SCHARFETTER, C., WINOKUR, G. *et al* (1988) Familial syndrome patterns in schizophrenia, schizoaffective disorder, mania and depression. *European Archives of Psychiatry and Neurological Sciences*, **237**, 115–123.

TSUANG, M. T., WINOKUR, G. & CROWE, R. R. (1980) Morbidity risks of schizophrenia and affective disorders among first degree relatives of patients with schizophrenia, mania, depression and surgical conditions. *British Journal of Psychiatry*, **137**, 497–504.

2 Critique of the concept of 'unitary psychosis'

SIR MARTIN ROTH

The concept of unitary psychosis was first advanced in the 19th century and is linked with the ideas of Griesinger (1845) and his contemporaries (Chapter 7). Griesinger's concept of '*Einheitspsychose*' (unitary psychosis) stemmed from a conviction that psychic diseases were brain diseases, a basic principle which could not be reconciled with classifications purely of symptoms. Although the concept of a unitary psychosis was to be rendered obsolete by the contributions of Kraepelin, Griesinger was an early pioneer of Kraepelin's attempts to establish psychiatry on empirical scientific foundations and to develop it as a branch of medicine with a special interest in cerebral physiology and pathology.

In the fifth edition of his textbook, Kraepelin (1896) expressed his unequivocal commitment to a medical conception of mental disease and iterated the main outlines of the classification in the eighth and final edition (1908–15). Dementia praecox was sharply differentiated from manic–depressive illness, which included 'melancholia'. The paranoid form of dementia praecox was differentiated from 'paraphrenia'. All psychoses were differentiated from neurotic and personality disorders, which were not recognised as diseases by Kraepelin or his followers.

Within a few decades of the publication of the fifth edition the essential characteristics of the Kraepelinian system had been widely accepted and were applied in the leading centres of psychiatric practice and scholarship in most parts of the world. France was a conspicuous exception. The concepts of dementia praecox, and later of schizophrenia, failed to gain acceptance there and the situation remains unchanged to the present.

Kraepelin managed to prevail over his main opponents by his exceptional gifts and the wealth of his experience as a clinical observer. This was reflected in the richness and clarity of the descriptions of cases in all his writings and the immense body of clinical observations he had assembled to delineate and differentiate disorders and to describe their course and outcome. Kraepelin was aware that the distinctions he drew with seemingly sharp boundaries oversimplified matters, as does every system of categorical classification in common with all taxonomies, but he never accepted the concept of unitary psychosis as a valid alternative to his own scheme.

As the influence of Kraepelin's classification extended, the concept of unitary psychosis was jettisoned in most centres of psychiatric thought. The validity of Kraepelin's clinical observations and concepts could be readily submitted to tests and they opened up fresh paths for scientific inquiry.

The successes achieved during the last half century through the application of neurobiological methods to problems of causation and treatment of psychiatric disorders have emanated to a considerable extent from Kraepelin's classification of psychiatric disorders. Pharmacology began with the discovery of the remarkable antipsychotic effects of chlorpromazine by Delay & Deniker (1952), the antischizophrenic properties of reserpine by Kline (1954), the antidepressant action of the monoamine oxidase inhibitor iproniazid by Crane & Kline in 1957 (Kline, 1958), and the antidepressant effects of imipramine by Kuhn (1957). Cade (1949) had described the efficacy of lithium in mania, but it was in the mid-1960s that it achieved general recognition. It is open to question whether the efficacy of any of these drugs would have come to light had they been submitted to therapeutic trials in groups of patients that included any and every form of psychosis had been admitted. Yet, in the light of the unitary-psychosis theory, there would have been no logical basis for excluding or indeed for identifying any subgroups. The onus is on those who would wish to introduce a unitary classification to prove that it is superior to the Kraepelinian system for the purposes of scientific investigation and for deciding on treatment and judging prognosis in clinical practice.

Differentiation of clinical features of schizophrenic and affective psychoses

One line of evidence that has been drawn upon to question the validity of the binary concept of the affective and schizophrenic psychoses has been derived from statistical analysis of the distribution of the summated symptom scores of a large sample of patients diagnosed as suffering from schizophrenic or affective psychosis. The investigations by Kendell & Gourlay (1970) have been quoted as having shown that the symptom profiles of the two disorders merge insensibly with each other. Their investigation of patients with schizophrenia and with affective disorder is described in Chapter 1 (p. 5). Examination of the distribution of the summated weights of the clinical features derived from discriminant function analysis has been interpreted by the authors as calling into question the binary hypothesis.

However, in Figure 1 of their paper (reproduced in Fig. 1.1, p. 5), the great majority of the patients fall into two distinct, clearly separated modes corresponding to the schizophrenic and affective groups. This interpretation was confirmed by the finding that the overall distribution of scores differed highly significantly from a normal distribution ($P < 0.001$). The authors describe this as a trimodal curve. The third mode, created by less than 10% of the patients, provides no valid basis for discounting the result that shows the curve departs significantly from a normal distribution. In a further sample of 128 patients with schizophrenia or affective psychosis they obtained a unimodal distribution, and inferred that the previous "trimodal" distribution may have been a "chance finding" (Brockington *et al*, 1979).

The evidence from course and outcome

Kendell & Brockington (1980) returned to the problem of continuity between schizophrenic and affective psychoses. They could find no evidence of a non-linear relationship between symptoms and outcome measures. Examination of the data calls into question the validity of this conclusion. Their 127 patients were divided into ten subgroups according to their score on the linear function that represented outcome. Some clear discontinuity seems to be manifest between the two sets of five subgroups, particularly in respect of the symptom measures of outcome, which had smaller standard deviations (Fig. 1.7, p. 12). In respect of their schizoaffective series, in two of the three measures discontinuity appeared to be present although the standard deviations were too large for firm conclusions (Figure 5 in Kendell & Brockington (1980)).

Studies of outcome of many forms of psychiatric disorder have repeatedly shown variables delineating pre-morbid personality, occupational and marital adjustment to make a contribution to the variance in respect of outcome, which is as large as or larger than that attributable to presenting symptoms and signs. There are very few such items in the original 38 variables subjected to discriminant functional analysis by Kendell & Gourlay (1970).

Long-term prospective follow-up studies are therefore required to determine the outcome of manic–depressive, schizophrenic and schizoaffective groups of patients selected by pre-defined criteria to determine their status in respect of clinical profile, hospital admission record, social and occupational adjustment, place of residence (at home, in hostel or in hospital) and adjustment in terms of family and other interpersonal relationships. However, the claim that there is no essential difference in outcome between schizophrenic and affective psychoses can already be called into question on the strength of hospital residence rates and a wide consensus of clinical opinion. Studies have shown that the prognosis of psychotic and endogenous affective disorders is not as favourable as had been believed in the past. Over

15–18 years, patients with endogenous as well as neurotic depressions had suffered repeated and at times lengthy relapses, often requiring admission (Lee & Murray, 1988; Kiloh *et al*, 1988). However, the evidence available shows that, in the long term, the prognosis of schizophrenia is far worse than this. If those with dementing disorders in old age are excluded from consideration, schizophrenics are by far the largest group among patients in the long-stay wards of mental hospitals, in community hostels for psychiatric patients, and among the homeless in the cities. Those with chronic depression or mania are rare exceptions.

Nor is there any evidence that the typical picture of deterioration in chronic schizophrenia also evolves in the chronic bipolar and unipolar psychoses. Blunting and impoverishment of affect, chronic delusions and hallucinations with an impenetrable incoherence of thought and speech, neologisms and stereotypies, autism, inertia, degradation of behaviour, severance of interpersonal relationships and social isolation do not occur among those in whom a diagnosis of manic–depressive or bipolar psychosis has been established by comprehensive evaluation at the outset.

From a phenomenological point of view, schizophrenia cannot be regarded as the more severe form of a unitary disorder of which manic–depressive psychosis is the more mild and benign version. There is no milder form of the great majority of the features of chronic schizophrenia cited among those with relapsing or chronic manic–depressive illness. Recent data provide no valid foundation for calling into question Kraepelin's original finding that the two main groups of psychoses were separated by differences in outcome as well as in respect of their severity and their quality.

The evidence from heredity

There is an increased prevalence of affective disorder among the first-degree relatives of those with schizophrenia, and also a raised prevalence of schizophrenia among the first-degree relatives of those with affective disorder (Slater, 1938, 1953; Powell *et al*, 1973). However, some allowance has to be made for the fact that the diagnosis of secondary cases is often made indirectly and that evidence derived from other members of the family and from case records is less reliable than personal interview and examination. Secondly, minor psychiatric disorder and depression in particular are to be found at high prevalence in the normal population. Excessive importance is liable to be attached to subclinical forms of such conditions and to certain personality disorders when discovered within pedigrees in which there are indubitably psychotic cases. Further, the DSM–III diagnosis of major depressive disorder is a weak and non-specific diagnostic concept (Strömgren, 1982). Thirdly, although a predisposition to a certain psychotic disorder may remain dormant in a substantial proportion of cases (penetrance of the genes responsible for the common forms of both schizophrenia and manic–depressive disorder being rather low), it may become manifest when this hereditary predisposition to mental disorder is associated with a coexistent latent predisposition for a different disorder. There is evidence, for example, that the spouse of the parent who carries the genes expressed as schizophrenia in a pedigree, makes an independent contribution through genetic factors or environmental influences, or both, to the psychopathology manifest in the children of the marriage (Kay *et al*, 1975; Stephens *et al*, 1976). These findings in the Newcastle schizophrenia study have been confirmed by the observations of Fowler (1975; Fowler & Cadoret, 1977) and similar observations were made in the course of the Danish–American adoption studies (Rosenthal, 1974).

Recent investigations with techniques of modern molecular genetics have shed light upon the 'unitary psychosis' problem. The inquiries have focused on those relatively rare forms of manic–depressive illness and schizophrenia in which the psychosis appeared from the pedigree to have been transmitted by a single Mendelian autosomal gene of dominant type, usually with high penetrance.

Working with a number of families among the Amish religious community in Pennsylvania, Egeland *et al* (1987) succeeded with the aid of two markers in mapping the gene for affective psychosis in these families to the tip of the short arm of chromosome 11. In another inquiry in Israel, five families comprising 161 individuals, 47 with bipolar or other affective disorder, were studied. The markers for colour blindness and G6PD deficiency were used. This study (Baron *et al*, 1987) established linkage with the putative gene for schizophrenia on an X-chromosome. Another investigation (Mendlewicz *et al*, 1987) mapped the responsible gene in ten families to a different locus on the X-chromosome.

Each of these findings has been called into question by attempts at replication. In the case of bipolar affective disorder in the kindred of Amish index cases, the initial positive lod score (which expresses the probability of linkage) of 4.08 reported by Egeland *et al* (1987) declined as the pedigree was extended. The last score for the 11p marker has been reported as − 9.31 (Kelso *et al*, 1989). Although there are rare pedigrees of bipolar disorder which are suggestive of autosomal dominant inheritance, none of the purported single genes held responsible for transmission of the disease has been conclusively mapped to a specific locus by linkage methods; none of the loci identified by linkage techniques has been independently corroborated.

Similar developments have been recorded in relation to schizophrenia. Bassett *et al* (1988) observed that two members of a Chinese family with schizophrenia shared a number of physical abnormalities as well as distinctive facial features not found in other members of the family. Cytogenetic investigation revealed translocation of part of chromosome 5 in both cases. The authors suggested that part of chromosome 5 may be the site of the gene that predisposes to schizophrenia. This stimulated attempts to test the prediction implied by this finding. Inquiries in seven families from Iceland and England (Sherrington *et al*, 1988) showed that linkage was probable between two probes and the 5q11–13 segment of chromosome 5 defined by Bassett *et al* as the possible site of the gene responsible for schizophrenia. It is interesting that the lod scores were increased when schizoid personality and certain minor psychiatric disorders were included in the calculations. Here again the results have been called into question by the negative findings of two groups (Kennedy *et al*, 1988; St Clair *et al*, 1989).

It is worthy of note that in no instance was a patient with a typical schizophrenic psychosis found in a manic–depressive pedigree nor was the reverse finding recorded in any of the schizophrenic pedigrees. For the present, molecular genetics lends no support to the unitary-psychosis theory. However, some of the disparities between the findings of different investigators may arise from the fact that, as in the case of many heritable neurological disorders, several different mutations may cause a similar phenotype (Roth, 1948).

Concordance by sex in paternally transmitted schizophrenia among male sibling pairs

Attention has been drawn by several authors to the fact that siblings with psychosis are more likely to be of the same sex than could be expected by chance. Crow (1988; Crow *et al*, 1989) has suggested a possible genetic explanation for this phenomenon. He has adduced evidence for the hypothesis that the major dominant gene responsible for the transmission of schizophrenia and also other psychotic disorders may be in the 'pseudo-autosomal' region of the X chromosomes. This refers to the distal segment of the short arms of these chromosomes in which there is cross-over, and therefore genetic exchange between the X and Y chromosomes during meiosis. As there has been evidence for autosomal transmission of both schizophrenic and affective psychoses, sex-linked transmission of these disorders has been regarded as unlikely in the past. However, as the gene in the pseudo-autosomal region would be transmitted in an apparently autosomal manner, the hypothesis suggested by Crow has not been refuted.

The gene would be passed above chance expectation to children of the same sex and inherited predominantly from the male parent. In an investigation of 120 families with at least one sibling pair concordant for schizophrenia it was found that affected members were significantly more often of the same sex when the history of schizophrenic illness was on the paternal side than when it was on the maternal side. The ratio of concordant to mixed-sex pairs with schizophrenia who had descended from a male parent in these families was three to one (Crow *et al*, 1989).

Crow (p. 43 and Table 3.4) summarises evidence for the presence of a similar phenomenon in the case of affective disorder (see also Crow 1989, 1990). In many previous investigations an excess of same-sex pairs as compared with opposite-sex pairs has been reported. However, there is an excess of female–female pairs which cannot be explained in terms of a pseudo-autosomal locus. Crow (1990) speculates that one and the same autosomal gene is likely to be responsible for same-sex concordance both in schizophrenic sibs and manic–depressive sibs although probable transmission through the male parent has been established only in the case of the former.

Alternative, more simple explanations for same-sex concordance have to be considered. The later age of onset and better prognosis of schizophrenic illness in women than men would be expected to give rise to some sex concordance along the following lines. In the case of males predisposed to schizophrenia, the age of onset of first illness would be in the second or third decade in the majority of cases, whereas female members of the same sibship who are also predisposed would be more likely to develop a first attack at a later age. Same-sex siblings are therefore liable to break down at about the same time, giving rise to 'same-sex concordance', with males being the more readily detected. The presence of a genetic predisposition to schizophrenia among women in the same sibship might be further concealed by their more favourable prognosis, so that the disorder is not only manifest at a later age but in a more benign and ambiguous form, or not at all. Moreover, in some women predisposed to schizophrenia the disease makes its first appearance in the form of paraphrenia or paranoid psychoses in middle or late life. Evidence for the genetic kinship of this disorder with schizophrenia has been presented by Kay (1959). Such a predisposition to illness may still be latent at the time of an inquiry into same-sex concordance and the psychosis manifest in old age would have been likely in the past to have been attributed to cerebral degeneration.

A similar effect might have arisen from the earlier age of onset and higher overall prevalence of manic–depressive disorders in women. The expected result would be an excess of female–female pairs in contrast to male–male sib concordance found in schizophrenia. This is in fact the pattern observed, so that the concordance patterns among affected sibs in both psychoses receive a hypothetical explanation in terms of sex-related differences in age of onset of each of the psychoses. It should be possible to design inquiries to determine whether the prevalence of same-sex concordance can be accounted for along the lines suggested here. The ingenious hypothesis which postulates a locus on the short arms of the X and Y chromosomes within the pseudo-autosomal region (where recombination takes place in male meiosis) as the site of the gene that predisposes to psychosis requires further investigation of this region with the aid of linkage methods in families that contain several psychotic patients. The relevance of Crow's theory for unitary psychosis resides in his dimensional model of psychotic disorder. The effects produced by the responsible pseudo-autosomal gene can be plotted on a continuum, with unipolar depression at one extreme and chronic schizophrenia at the other.

Schizoaffective disorder

The early decades of this century saw the delineation of a number of disorders which seemed to cut across the Kraepelinian entities. These were the important contributions of Jaspers (1913), Kretschmer (1918) and Wimmer (1916), among others, to the concept of 'psychogenic psychosis'. They are relevant to the general theme of this chapter in that they not only impute a psychogenic cause for certain psychoses that would be regarded as wholly 'endogenous' by traditional psychiatrists, but some of these disorders are depressive, others predominantly paranoid or quasi-schizophrenic in type, and others still exhibit features of both these groups of disorders (Kasanin, 1933; Staehelin, 1946; Leonhard, 1957). However, the clinical characteristics and aetiological origins of these disorders remain controversial.

In the 1930s, a group of papers was devoted to disorders that appeared to establish lines of continuity between schizophrenic and closely related psychoses on the one hand and manic–depressive disorders on the other. They included schizoaffective psychosis (Kasanin, 1933), schizophreniform psychosis (Langfeldt, 1937) and, later, cycloid psychosis (Leonhard, 1957). All of these can be regarded broadly speaking as 'schizoaffective' disorders.

The increasing tendency to make a diagnosis of schizoaffective disorder has probably arisen in part from the nature of the criteria laid down in DSM–III–R for the diagnosis of this condition (American Psychiatric Association, 1987). For example, the patient who exhibits mood-incongruent psychotic symptoms has to be diagnosed as suffering from major affective disorder provided the incongruent delusional symptoms have never occurred in the absence of affective symptoms. In the presence of passivity feelings, 'primary' delusions or delusions of thought withdrawal or other 'nuclear' features, the validity of this criterion is open to question. Further, patients with typical episodes of mania or depression have to be judged as schizophrenic if the affective symptoms develop after those suggestive of schizophrenia. It would be more appropriate for the earlier diagnosis to be reconsidered. Such patients are likely to be given a diagnosis of schizoaffective disorder, but an experienced clinician working with less rigid diagnostic rules may, after thorough examination, feel justified in rejecting the earlier diagnosis.

In some studies a single mood-incongruent delusion or first-rank symptom qualifies patients for a diagnosis of schizoaffective disorder. This draws excessively sharp lines of demarcation around affective disorder. No single symptom deserves to be accorded such decisive importance.

Some investigators regard schizoaffective disorder as a distinct group of psychoses intermediate between the two other major psychotic disorders, rather than as a blend of two existent disorders. This is improbable, since among the first-degree relatives of those with schizoaffective disorder, it is schizophrenic illness or affective psychosis alone or both of these psychoses that predominate in the same pedigree, and not schizoaffective disorder. For example, in the study of Angst *et al* (1979) the majority of diagnosed first-degree relatives of schizoaffective patients were either schizophrenic (5.2% of total) or affective psychotic (6.6%). Only a small proportion (3% of total) were given a diagnosis of schizoaffective disorder, which was broadly defined. Schizoaffective disorder is therefore transmitted only to about a fifth of those offspring of patients who develop a psychosis. In the next generation it mostly segregates into one or other of the traditional major psychoses.

Another possible origin for the affective component of some patients with schizoaffective disorder has been brought to light. In the genetic investigations of schizophrenia it is often implicitly assumed that mating has occurred at random. But there is evidence for assortative mating from the personalities of spouses of individuals predisposed to schizophrenic illness (Stephens *et al*, 1975; Kay *et al*, 1975). In an investigation of psychotic families and controls it was found that abnormal sibs were concentrated in the families with abnormal fathers. Moreover, female siblings appeared to be relatively immune from the psychopathology of either parent, as reflected in the low prevalence of abnormal personalities among females and their early marriages. In the families of schizophrenic probands, the fathers of male siblings with personality disorder were often markedly abnormal, their personalities being characterised by psychopathy, heavy drinking or a record of criminality. They often abandoned the mother of the family. Abnormal personalities in the male siblings may therefore have been derived from polygenic factors and adverse environmental influences emanating from the non-schizophrenic or non-schizoid parent. Similar findings have been published by Fowler & Cadoret (1977) and Rosenthal (1974). Those sibs of the proband who develop personality disorder would also have been at risk for the development of affective disorders. The depressive disorders of psychopaths are listed in a number of classifications of affective disorder (Paykel, 1971), and the depressive states and suicides of those with psychopathy have in recent years been manifest in the growing phenomenon of gaol suicides.

To the extent that some cases of schizoaffective disorder may originate from the personality-disordered non-schizophrenic spouse of a schizophrenic parent, this disorder does not support the case for any continuum of *psychotic* disorders.

What is measured along the unitary-psychoticism continuum?

It is not clear what variable can be plotted along the abscissa of any graph that purports to represent the continuum of psychotic disorders. Crow (1986) has suggested a continuum extends "from uni-polar, through bi-polar affective illness and schizoaffective psychosis to typical schizophrenia, with increasing degrees of defect". Some forms of acute depressive illness may be much more severe in respect of the character of the behaviour disturbance manifest, the suffering experienced and the risk to life or actual mortality entailed than in cases of schizophrenic disorder. The same statement can be made about manic illness. In respect of liability to impoverishment of affect, inertia, withdrawal, deterioration of personal habits and loss of characteristic individual traits, a substantial proportion of schizophrenic patients are more severely affected. But no corresponding quantitatively graded change with any resemblance to this phenomenon evolves during the course of unipolar or bipolar affective psychosis. It is therefore inadmissible to interpret personality deterioration as a continuous measure of the severity of a unitary psychosis. Schizophrenia is set qualitatively apart by the progressive dismemberment of the personality (and the absence of any reliable predictors of this change) from the affective and related psychoses.

It has therefore to be asked what quantitative measures can be devised to estimate 'psychoticism' so as to assign a position on a unitary psychotic continuum to individual patients with psychosis. How is the validity of such measures to be assessed? By what other means can the hypothetical construct 'psychoticism' as a dimension common to all forms of affective and schizophrenic illness be validated by empirical observation? As the exponents of the concept of unitary psychosis have not provided answers to any of these questions they have failed to establish heuristic value for it.

Age of onset, course and treatment response

The fact that both psychoses may occur at any stage of adult life has been quoted as a feature they have in common (Crow, 1986), but the variation of incidence during different stages of the lifespan is markedly different in the two disorders. The peak incidence of schizophrenia is between the ages of 15 and 25 years. By the age of 35 years, 62% of the total risk has been survived in men and 47% in women; at 45 years the figures are 82% and 68% respectively (Slater & Roth, 1969). In contrast, in manic–depressive psychosis (Slater, 1938), at the age of 20 only 2% of the risk is survived and at 40 years 33%. The curve describing incidence rises at each age to a high plateau which is well maintained during the middle years. Even at 60 years 21% of the risk of developing manic–depressive illness remains. In schizophrenia the proportions of men and women who remain at risk are 2% and 6% respectively.

In depressive and manic psychosis the course is one of recurrent attacks, in most cases with periods of remission between. Personality does not deteriorate. In schizophrenia about a third of patients pursue a chronic course with personality deterioration. In a further third the course is recurrent, or a relapsing course is observed in a small proportion of cases. Complete remissions are uncommon in these cases. Residual deficits with personality decline that increases with successive attacks is a more common course of events.

Electroconvulsive treatment (ECT) is effective in some cases of schizophrenic psychosis but in a smaller proportion and in a more limited segment of the clinical picture than in depressive illness. The effects of ECT that discriminate between the psychoses are more numerous than those that are common to them. Tricyclic antidepressants and monoamine oxidase inhibitors, both of which are efficacious in depressive states (including endogenous disorders), have no effect or exacerbate the symptoms of schizophrenia. Neuroleptic substances will alleviate or promote a complete remission from the central features of schizophrenic disorders for months or longer. In contrast, in affective psychosis the effects are confined to epiphenomenal features of agitation, restlessness and to some extent insomnia. No evidence exists that neuroleptic substances can by themselves promote recovery that extends over the greater part of the range of symptoms and signs in depressive illness; used as the only form of treatment they also fail in a substantial proportion of patients with mania. Lithium carbonate has been reported to be of some value in a proportion of cases of schizoaffective disorder, although the data are conflicting. But there is no good evidence that it is effective in either the treatment or the prophylaxis of schizophrenic illness. Similarities of treatment response cannot therefore be invoked in evidence for a unitary concept.

Conclusions

The validity of the findings which have been interpreted to signify that the symptoms of the major psychoses merge without visible break is of doubtful validity. Moreover, there are independent lines of evidence that rebut the null hypothesis that only a single disorder is delineated by these distributions. The excess of patients with schizophrenic illness found in families of probands with bipolar disorder and to a lesser extent the reverse of this situation which has also been placed on record is open to other and more economical interpretations than that offered by the theory of unitary psychosis.

The concept of schizoaffective disorder, as a specific psychosis which bridges the divide between the two main independent psychoses, is not upheld. The offspring of such patients manifest schizophrenia in some cases, bipolar disorder in others; only a minority of such offspring manifest schizoaffective disorder. The nosological status, treatment response and course and outcome of the minority group of patients with schizoaffective disorder remains to be investigated.

The rare pedigrees in which schizophrenia or manic–depressive psychosis appears to be transmitted by an autosomal dominant gene (although attempts to map such a gene to a specific locus have failed for the present) have not provided any evidence for the concept of unitary psychosis. Although in each type of pedigree some first-degree relatives have been found to manifest other conditions, these have been non-specific minor affective or personality disorders. In no mainly schizophrenic pedigree has a single case of a bipolar or other affective psychosis been found. Nor have incongruous findings of this sort been recorded in pedigrees from which bipolar probands have been drawn.

Same-sex concordance between siblings with psychosis has been utilised by Crow as the basis of a specific aetiological explanation of a unitary psychosis. The phenomenon has been tentatively explained (Crow, 1988; Crow *et al*, 1989) with the aid of the hypothesis that the major dominant gene responsible for the transmission of schizophrenia and also other psychotic disorders may be in the 'pseudo-autosomal' region of the sex chromosomes. This ingenious hypothesis deserves further inquiry. An alternative explanation for the phenomenon of same-sex concordance between psychotic twins may be provided by the significant differences between the sexes in the age of onset of illness in each of the psychotic disorders. Crow considers that his 'psychotic gene' may be expressed in the form of any syndrome along the entire spectrum that extends from unipolar depression at one end of the continuum of psychosis to chronic schizophrenia at the other. The findings summarised in this chapter provide little evidence in favour of such versatility in expression of the gene (or genes) responsible for the transmission of schizophrenia or affective psychosis.

As no testable hypotheses regarding the aetiological origins of psychotic disorders, or the treatment or prediction of outcome, have emanated from it, the concepts of unitary psychosis and of a continuum of psychoses are of dubious heuristic value.

References

AMERICAN PSYCHIATRIC ASSOCIATION (1987) *Diagnostic and Statistical Manual of Mental Disorders* (3rd edn, revised) (DSM–III–R). Washington, DC: APA.

ANGST, J., FELDER, W. & LOHMEYER, B. (1979) Schizoaffective disorders: results of a genetic investigation. *Journal of Affective Disorders*, **1**, 139–155.

BARON, M., RISCH, N., HAMBURGER, R., *et al* (1987) Genetic linkage between X-chromosome markers and bipolar affective illness. *Nature*, **326**, 289–292.

BASSETT, A. S., McGILLIVRAY, B. C., JONES, B. D., *et al* (1988) Partial trisomy chromosome 5 cosegregating with schizophrenia. *Lancet*, **i**, 799–801.

BROCKINGTON, I. F., KENDELL, R. E., WAINWRIGHT, S., *et al* (1979) The distinction between the affective psychoses and schizophrenia. *British Journal of Psychiatry*, **135**, 243–248.

CADE, J. F. J. (1949) Lithium salts in treatment of psychotic excitement. *Medical Journal of Australia*, **ii**, 349.

CROW, T. J. (1986) The continuum of psychosis and its implication for the structure of the gene. *British Journal of Psychiatry*, **149**, 419–429.
—— (1988) Sex chromosomes and psychosis: the case for a pseudoautosomal locus. *British Journal of Psychiatry*, **153**, 675–683.
—— (1989) Pseudoautosomal locus for the cerebral dominance gene. *Lancet*, ii, 339–348.
—— (1990) The continuum of psychosis and its genetic origins. The sixty-fifth Maudsley lecture. *British Journal of Psychiatry*, **156**, 788–797.
——, DeLISI, L. E. & JOHNSTONE, E. C. (1989) Concordance by sex in sibling pairs with schizophrenia is paternally inherited: evidence for a pseudoautosomal locus. *British Journal of Psychiatry*, **155**, 92–97.
DELAY, J. & DENIKER, P. (1952) Cas de psychoses traités par la cure prolangee et continué de 4568 R.P. *Annales Medico-Psychologiques*, **110**, 364.
EGELAND, J. A., GERHARD, D. W., PAULS, D. L., *et al* (1987) Bipolar affective disorders linked to DNA markers on chromosome 11. *Nature*, **325**, 783–787.
FOWLER, R. C. (1975) Spouses of schizophrenics: a blind comparative study. *Comprehensive Psychiatry*, **16**, 346–359.
—— & CADORET, R. J. (1977) Psychiatric illness in the offspring of schizophrenics. *Comprehensive Psychiatry*, **16**, 339–342.
GRIESINGER, W. (1845) *Iber der Pathologie und Therapie der Geisteskranken.*(*Mental Pathology and Therapeutics* (1965). New York: Hafner.)
JASPERS, K. (1913) *General Psychopathology* (trans. (1963) J. Hoenig & M. W. Hamilton). Manchester: Manchester University Press.
KASANIN, J. (1933) The acute schizoaffective psychoses. *American Journal of Psychiatry*, **13**, 97–126.
KAY, D. W. K. (1959) Observations on the natural history and genetics of old age psychoses. *Proceedings of the Royal Society of Medicine*, **52**, 791–794.
——, ROTH, M., ATKINSON, M. W., *et al* (1975) Environmental and hereditary factors in the schizophrenias of old age ('late paraphrenia') and their bearing on general problems of causation in schizophrenia. *British Journal of Psychiatry*, **127**, 109–119.
KELSO, J. R., GINNS, E. I., EGELAND, J. A., *et al* (1989) Re-evaluation between chromosome 11P loci in the gene for bi-polar affective disorders in Old Order Amish. *Nature*, **342**, 238–243.
KENDELL, R. E. & GOURLAY, J. (1970) The clinical distinction between the affective psychoses and schizophrenia. *British Journal of Psychiatry*, **177**, 261–266.
—— & BROCKINGTON, I. F. (1980) The identification of disease entities and the relationship between schizophrenic and affective psychoses. *British Journal of Psychiatry*, **137**, 324–331.
KENNEDY, J. L., GUIFFRA, L. A., Moises, H. W., *et al* (1988) Evidence against linkage of schizophrenia to markers on chromosome 5 in a Northern Swedish pedigree. *Nature*, **336**, 167–170.
KILOH, L. G., ANDREWS, G. & NEILSON, R. M. (1988) The long-term outcome of depressive illness. *British Journal of Psychiatry*, **153**, 752–757.
KLINE, N. S. (1954) Use of rauwolfia serpentina benth in neuropsychiatric conditions. *Annals of the New York Academy of Science*, **59**, 107.
—— (1958) Clinical experience with iproniazid (Marsilid). *Journal of Clinical and Experimental Psychopathology*, **19** (suppl. 1), 72–78.
KRAEPELIN, E. (1896) *Psychiatrie, ein Lehrbuch fur Studierende und Arzte* (5th edn). Leipzig: Barth.
KRETSCHMER, E. (1918) *Der sensitive Beziehungswahn*. Berlin: Springer.
KUHN, R. (1957) Uber die Behandlung depressiver Zustaende mit einem Iminodibenzyl-derivat. *Schweizeerische Medizinische Wochenschrift*, **87**, 1135–1140.
LANGFELDT, G. (1937) The prognosis in schizophrenia and the factors influencing the course of the disease. *Acta Psychiatrica Scandinavica* (suppl. 13).
LEE, A. S. & MURRAY, R. M. (1988) The long-term outcome of Maudsley depressives. *British Journal of Psychiatry*, **153**, 741–751.
LEONHARD, K. (1957) *Aufteilung der endogenen Psychosen*. Berlin: Akademie Verlag.
MENDLEWICZ, J., SIMON, P., SEVY, S., *et al* (1987) Polymorphic DNA marker on X chromosome and manic depression. *Lancet*, i, 1230–1232.
PAYKEL, E. S. (1971) Classification of depressed patients: a cluster analysis derived grouping. *British Journal of Psychiatry*, **118**, 275–288.

POWELL, A., THOMSON, N., HALL, D. J., *et al* (1973) Parent–child concordance with respect to sex and diagnosis in schizophrenia and manic–depressive psychosis. *British Journal of Psychiatry*, **123**, 653–658.

ROSENTHAL, D. (1974) The concept of subschizophrenic disorders. In *Genetics, Environment and Psychopathology* (eds S. A. Mednick, F. Schulsinger, F. Higgins, *et al*). Oxford: North Holland.

ROTH, M. (1948) On a possible relationship between hereditary ataxia and peroneal atrophy. *Brain*, **71**, 416–433.

SHERRINGTON, R., BRYNJOLFSSON, J., PETURSSON, H., *et al* (1988) Localisation of a susceptibility locus for schizophrenia on chromosome 5. *Nature*, **335**, 164–167.

SLATER, E. (1938) Zur Erbpathologie des manisch–depressiven Irreseins. Die Eltern und Kinder von Manisch–Depressiven. *Z. Ges. Neurol. Psychiat.*, **163**, 1–47.

—— (1953) *Psychotic and Neurotic Illness in Twins*. Medical Research Council Special Report Series No. 278. London: MRC.

—— & ROTH, M. (1969) *Clinical Psychiatry*. London: Baillière, Tindall & Cassell.

STAEHELIN, J. E. (1946) Zur Frage der Emotionspsychosen. *Bulletin der Schwiezischen Akademie der Medizinischen Wissenschaften*, **2**, 121–130.

ST CLAIR, D., BLACKWOOD, D., MUIR, W., *et al* (1989) No linkage of chromosome 5q 11–13 markers to schizophrenia in Scottish families. *Nature*, **340**, 391–393.

STEPHENS, D. A., ATKINSON, M. W., KAY, D. W. K., *et al* (1975) Psychiatric morbidity in parents and sibs of schizophrenics and non-schizophrenics. *British Journal of Psychiatry*, **127**, 97–108.

——, ——, ——, *et al* (1976) Psychiatric morbidity in parents and sibs of schizophrenics and non-schizophrenics. *British Journal of Psychiatry*, **127**, 97–108.

STRÖMGREN, E. (1982) The strengths and weaknesses of DSM–III. In *International Perspectives on DSM–III* (eds R. L. Spitzer, J. B. W. Williams & A. E. Skodol). Washington, DC: APA.

WIMMER, A. (1916) *Psykogene Sindssygdomsformer* ['Psychogenic varieties of mental diseases'] *in St. Hans Hospital 1816–1916. Jubilee Publication*. Copenhagen: Gad.

3 The failure of the Kraepelinian binary concept and the search for the psychosis gene

TIMOTHY J. CROW

The argument of this chapter is that the psychoses, rather than representing the two major disease entities of the Kraepelinian system, or the single but variable unitary psychosis that Kraepelin's system superseded, constitute a continuum. Such a continuum of psychotic illnesses could encompass variations within as well as between the affective and schizophrenic realms.

Emil Kraepelin's key contribution was to establish that there is a relationship between the form of a psychotic illness and its outcome. Illnesses in which affective change is a prominent component have a better outcome than those in which affective features are less prominent and in which the psychotic phenomena cannot be understood as secondary to affective change. The success of the Kraepelinian system, even its survival, owes everything to the reality of this relationship. Yet the independence of the two Kraepelinian entities has never been satisfactorily established (and Kraepelin himself had doubts). Notwithstanding, the influence of the Kraepelinian concept is pervasive: every textbook has separate chapters on schizophrenia and affective disorder. A major objective of operational diagnostic criteria such as the Research Diagnostic Criteria (RDC; Spitzer et al, 1978) and DSM–III (American Psychiatric Association, 1980) is to separate these two entities with maximum reliability.

The assumption underlying such endeavours – that affective disorder and schizophrenia have different underlying pathogeneses and aetiology – has been paralytic to our thinking and stultifying to research. It obscures some general relationships that encompass both affective and schizophrenic psychoses and may provide a clue to aetiology: both types of psychosis have an onset within the reproductive epoch, and an incidence that is worldwide and without established relation to environmental or cultural variables.

If, as seems increasingly likely, the psychoses are genetic in origin, our most urgent task is to identify the locus. The Kraepelinian binary concept generates the expectation that there are at least two loci; the concept of a continuum leads to the prediction that there is but a single locus. It is argued here that one particular site in the genome is compatible with established observations on familial clustering, and can explain some other enigmas.

Do family studies support the Kraepelinian separation?

Until recently the challenge to the Kraepelinian system has come from a small band of workers with interests in fields other than genetics. Thus, for example, Kendell (1987) has approached the problem through phenomenology and nosology, Menninger *et al* (1958) and Beck (1972) have been interested in therapeutic strategies, and Flor-Henry (1983) in neuropsychology. Almost without exception those who have relied upon family studies (e.g. G. Winokur, E. S. Gershon, R. Cloninger, K. S. Kendler) have followed Kraepelin in adopting a binary view. Karlsson (1974) applied a global concept of psychosis to the historical records in Iceland. Only Angst, with an early interest in schizoaffective psychoses, has adopted a position of relative agnosticism. An order of battle (Fig. 3.1) illustrates the predilection of geneticists for the Kraepelinian viewpoint and the diversity of interests of the protagonists of the continuum viewpoint.

At first sight it appears ominous for the continuum concept that those who have been most concerned with the genetic basis, who might therefore be expected to be the most hard-headed and quantitative, have been the strongest advocates of the Kraepelinian position. Thus Gershon & Rieder (1980) wrote that "evidence from twin and family studies suggests that bipolar manic–depressive illness and chronic schizophrenia are distinct entities". According to Reich *et al* (1982) "the genetic diathesis for affective disorders is independent of that for other psychiatric disorders" and Loranger (1981), on the basis of a family study using DSM–III criteria, concluded that "manic–depression and schizophrenia are genetically unrelated diseases".

Part at least of the confidence that genetic researchers have had in the Kraepelinian concept is based upon the fallacy of the excluded middle. Thus such studies are almost invariably conducted upon samples which are

Binary theorists		Continuum theorists
Kraepelin		
Winokur		Menninger
		Kendell
		Beck
		Karlsson
	Angst	
Gershon		
Kendler		
		Flor-Henry
Cloninger		
		Crow

Fig. 3.1. Protagonists of the binary and continuum theories as judged from published contributions up to 1986

'purified' (as in Loranger's study) so that they include only probands who meet standard criteria for either classic Kraepelinian affective disorder or schizophrenia. Schizoaffective or atypical cases are excluded, and the conclusion drawn is that there is relatively little overlap in family studies between the psychoses. Such a strategy is clearly inadequate to demonstrate the bimodality that is assumed in the Kraepelinian two-entities principle. Some workers have come to realise that the intermediate psychoses raise real problems for the binary system; others have yet to appreciate the difficulties presented by recent studies even, in some cases, where these are their own (see pp. 36–39). As Kendell points out in Chapter 1 (p. 2), Kraepelin himself was aware of the problem. In one of his last contributions (Kraepelin, 1920) he wrote: "Perhaps it is also possible to tackle the difficulties which prevent us from distinguishing reliably between manic–depressive insanity and dementia praecox . . . it is becoming increasingly clear that we cannot distinguish satisfactorily between these two illnesses. . . ."

In family studies what is required to test the two-entities principle is a sample of probands that includes a representative selection of both typical states and intermediate psychoses. The question to be asked is whether the distribution of illness in relatives is or is not bimodal along the axis that separates the typical syndromes. Bimodality supports the two-entities principle, failure to find it in a suitably selected sample favours the continuum concept.

Ødegård (1972) was perhaps the first to mount such an investigation. In a series of consecutive admissions with psychosis to the Oslo mental hospitals, he included schizophrenic psychoses with three grades of defect, and reactive, atypical affective and typical manic–depressive psychoses, in his classification of probands. In this typology it is likely that those illnesses which in other systems would be described as schizoaffective will be included in the category of schizophrenia without defect, or, 'reactive' or 'atypical affective' psychoses. Illnesses in first-degree and second-degree relatives are classified into the three categories of 'schizophrenia', and 'reactive' and 'affective' psychoses. When illness in the proband is arranged along a continuum, the proportion of ill relatives in each of these categories can be examined (Fig. 3.2). The proportion suffering from schizophrenia is largest among the relatives of probands with schizophrenia with severe defect and declines progressively across the continuum, as the proportion of relatives with affective disorder rises. The proportion with reactive psychosis is highest in the relatives of probands with that diagnosis and declines in either direction from this point to minima at the pure-defect and manic–depressive extremes.

The findings are more readily assimilated to a continuum than to a binary concept. At each point on the proband diagnostic scale there is overlap with adjacent categories. The intermediate classes of psychosis do not form discrete and separate entities; rather they appear to have clear and quantitatively varying relationships with the prototypical symptom patterns. Of particular

34   *Crow*

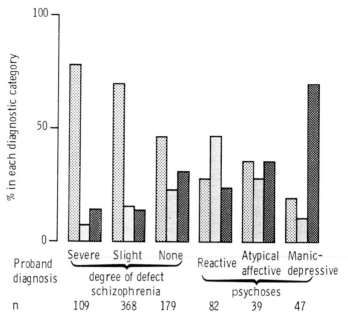

Fig. 3.2. Relative risks of psychiatric disorder (▨ schizophrenia, ▨ reactive psychosis, ▨ affective psychosis), classified from case histories, in the first-degree and second-degree relatives of a consecutive series of admissions of patients with psychosis (data taken from Ødegård, 1972)

interest is the fact that within the three categories of schizophrenic illness the proportion of illnesses among the relatives that are schizophrenic declines while those that are affective increases as the severity of defect in the proband changes from severe to slight to absent. Similar relationships between form of illness in the proband and the presence of affective disorder in the relatives were reported by Kant (1942) in a study of recovered and deteriorated schizophrenic patients. It is unclear why this should be the case if schizophrenia and affective illness are genetically unrelated.

Similar findings on the spectrum of psychotic illness are reported by Angst and his colleagues from Zurich. These workers started with the question of whether schizoaffective disorders are related to affective or to schizophrenic illness (Angst *et al*, 1979) and later extended the scope of their inquiries to include the prototypical syndromes. In a recent analysis (Table 3.1) their findings are presented with probands classified as having unipolar and bipolar affective disorder, schizoaffective illness of a predominantly affective or of a predominantly schizophrenic type, and schizophrenia. Relatives were classified into the categories of schizophrenia and affective disorder. As in Ødegård's study, the ratio of schizophrenic to affective relatives increases across the spectrum from unipolar illness to typical schizophrenia.

In an earlier report, Angst *et al* (1983) had written:

TABLE 3.1
Morbid risk in first-degree relatives

	Unipolar	Bipolar	Schizoaffective disorder (predominantly affective)	Schizoaffective disorder (predominantly schizophrenic)	Schizophrenia
No. of probands	58	31	34	35	105
No. of affected relatives with					
schizophrenia	10	4	19	18	31
affective psychoses	24	6	14	4	5
Ratio of schizophrenic to affective relatives (age-corrected)	0.30	0.47	0.92	2.99	5.05

Data from Angst & Scharfetter (1990).

"The obtained results are certainly puzzling in certain aspects. The underlying hypothesis of a continuum of psychosis is not disproved by our results. They show that on a descriptive level of symptoms and syndromes, taking into account the whole course of a psychosis, the dichotomy into schizophrenia and affective disorders is highly questionable. We do not only find transitional groups but also marked affective symptomatology underlying or superimposed to schizoprenia. . . . Based on our findings, we do not conclude that a unitary psychosis exists but we think of a continuum of psychopathological subgroups with a lot of overlap which may also differ to a certain extent in other respects such as course, genetics and response to treatment."

In their later discussions these authors write that "our analyses reveal no clear breeding true of either affective disorders or schizophrenia" (Stassen *et al*, 1988) and "The group of schizobipolar patients survives despite all attempts to break them down and to allocate them to schizophrenia and to affective disorder" (Angst & Scharfetter, 1990).

A further indicator of a sea-change in the literature comes from the studies of Gershon and colleagues at the National Institute of Mental Health (NIMH). Whereas Gershon & Rieder (1980) concluded that mania and schizophrenia could be considered as distinct genetic entities, subsequent work significantly modified this view. Thus, in a family study of affective and schizoaffective probands, Gershon *et al* (1982) concluded the data were compatible with the different affective disorders representing thresholds on a continuum that extends from unipolar, through bipolar I and bipolar II, to schizoaffective illness "representing greatest vulnerability"; and in a study of the relatives of patients with chronic psychosis (schizophrenia or schizoaffective disorder), Gershon *et al* (1988) found there was no tendency for schizoaffective diagnosis or acute psychoses to aggregate separately from schizophrenia. Increased incidence of affective disorder (bipolar plus unipolar) was found in the relatives of patients with both schizoaffective disorder and schizophrenia. Gershon *et al* (1988) considered a number of possible interpretations and concluded that:

"there is much evidence suggesting that there must be at least graduations of affectivity and schizophrenicity. Presence of schizoaffective disorder in relatives, for example, is more associated with schizophrenic probands than with probands with chronic schizoaffective disorder. . . . Patients with schizoaffective disorder have more relatives with bipolar disorder than do schizophrenic patients. Studied by the same methods, patients with affective disorders have a lower incidence of psychosis . . . in their relatives than do the patients with schizophrenia or chronic schizoaffective disorder."

The most recent contribution is that of Maier *et al* (1989), who studied 450 probands with affective, schizoaffective and schizophrenic psychoses. A total of 1250 first-degree relatives were interviewed with the Schedule for Affective Disorders and Schizophrenia, lifetime version, supplemented by interviews for polydiagnostic classification and personality disorders. In general agreement with a continuum concept, these authors found that "the familial pattern of disorders found is characterised by an unspecificity of diagnostic entities". Further analyses of this large and systematic investigation will be of considerable interest.

Thus support for the Kraepelinian position is somewhat less than as represented in Fig. 3.1. Kraepelin's adherence to the two-entities principle was conditioned by reservations. Angst has moved from a position of agnosticism towards the continuum viewpoint and Gershon, on the basis of the studies that he and his colleagues have carried out at NIMH, has switched from adherence to the classic two-entities principle to the view that no clear lines can be drawn – that is, to a version of the continuum concept (Fig. 3.3).

The case of the 'palaeo-Kraepelinians'

Three strong protagonists of the binary concept remain – Cloninger, Kendler and Winokur. Their views and the evidence that they use to support them deserve careful consideration.

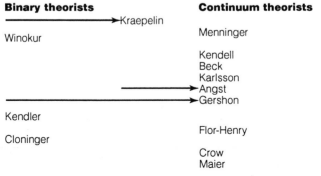

Fig. 3.3. Adherence to the binary and continuum theories as in 1990

Cloninger *et al* (1985) conducted the only study so far to challenge the conclusion of Kendell & Brockington (1980) that no bimodal separation of the prototypical psychoses can be achieved on the basis of phenomenology or outcome (see Chapter 1, and Fig. 1.5, p. 9). Their constellation of four features (persecutory delusions, delusions of control, firmly fixed mood-incongruent delusions, and auditory hallucinations) (minus one for the presence of a history of spending sprees plus elation) was used to demonstrate a bimodal separation of schizophrenic patients defined by the Feighner criteria from other subjects. The authors claim that not only did their scale identify 68% of schizophrenics and achieve separation from other subjects but that it was also useful for predicting outcome and the presence of a similar syndrome in relatives. A number of points are relevant (a–c).

(a) The strategy adopted identifies a concept of schizophrenia that is notably restricted. The Feighner criteria require a history of six months of continuous illness, and exclude a large number of patients who by other criteria (e.g. the Research Diagnostic Criteria, and CATEGO system) will be classified as schizophrenic. Yet by the Cloninger criterion 32% even of the Feighner-positive schizophrenic patients will be excluded. Therefore if, as the authors claim, these patients form a separate group of psychotic illnesses (possibly 'true Kraepelinian schizophrenia') it is not one that corresponds to many other concepts of the extent and frequency of the disease. Many non-affective, non-schizophrenic psychoses remain to be accounted for.

(b) The family-history part of the study is not a critical test of bimodality. The fact that schizophrenic illnesses are found more commonly among the relatives of probands with typical schizophrenic illnesses than among those of probands with affective and other psychoses and normal individuals is the generally accepted finding. The question to be addressed is whether accepting the definition Cloninger *et al* propose for schizophrenia allows one to identify families that include an excess of individuals with schizophrenia but no excess of schizoaffective or atypical psychoses. The findings of Gershon *et al* (1988) and Angst & Scharfetter (1990) suggest that this will not be the case.

(c) An index of absence of affective disorder (history of spending sprees with marked elation) is used to identify the group of 'true' schizophrenics. It would be interesting to know how much the findings depend upon this. Perhaps it is another indication of the way in which the propensity for affective change diminishes as severity of schizophrenia increases along the psychotic continuum.

For each of these reasons the Cloninger study remains indecisive. If bimodality has been established, the region of rarity is located far to the right (i.e. the schizophrenic extreme) on the line along which affective disorder and schizophrenia are separated. If this definition of schizophrenia is substantiated many psychoses hitherto labelled schizophrenic will require a new name.

A notable illustration of the relevance of atypical psychoses and of the bias introduced by sampling as probands only those patients who suffer from classic affective and schizophrenic psychoses is provided by Kendler *et al* (1986). Whereas previously Kendler and colleagues had applied DSM–III criteria for affective disorder and schizophrenia to the Iowa 500 series of patients and controls and their relatives, and had concluded that the Kraepelinian separation was generally supported, in this study they examined a series of probands with a chart diagnosis of schizophrenia who did not meet the Feighner criteria. These individuals were allocated to the DSM–III diagnostic categories of schizophreniform disorder, schizoaffective disorder and psychotic affective illness. Kendler *et al*'s conclusions deserve full quotation:

> "The pattern of psychopathology in relatives of schizophreniform probands closely resembled that found previously in relatives of schizophrenic probands. Relatives of schizoaffective probands had an excess risk for schizophrenia, other psychoses, and bipolar illness. The pattern of illness found in relatives of probands meeting Research Diagnostic Criteria for mainly schizophrenic schizoaffective disorder appeared indistinguishable from that of relatives of schizophrenic probands. Relatives of probands with psychotic affective disorder had an excess risk for schizophrenia and for unipolar and bipolar affective disorder." (Kendler *et al*, 1986)

It is instructive to examine these conclusions in an attempt to determine where the dividing line between schizophrenia and affective disorder might be drawn. Firstly, since the spectrum of symptoms in the schizophreniform disorders is the same as in schizophrenia while their duration is less, the similarity in genetic relationships is to be expected. However, in that some of these schizophreniform illnesses (and also the DSM–III schizophrenia cases) are unlikely to meet the Cloninger criterion of true schizophrenia, the overlap here is an embarrassment for Cloninger *et al*'s definition. Secondly, the finding that the relatives of patients with schizoaffective psychoses have an excess risk for both schizophrenia and affective illness is problematic for the Kraepelinian viewpoint unless these psychoses can be subdivided into schizophrenic and affective subtypes. But this the studies of Angst and co-workers have failed to establish – no such distinction can be justified. Lastly, the findings in the relatives of patients with psychotic affective disorder in this series suggest a greater overlap between the prototypical psychoses than was apparent in the earlier DSM–III-based studies on the Iowa series.

Overall the findings give no comfort to the Kraepelinian concept. The impact on Kendler's own thinking is interesting to follow. Previously, in collaboration with Hays (Kendler & Hays, 1983), he had studied patients with schizophrenia defined by DSM–III criteria and had identified a group of 28 with a first-degree relative with affective disorder. These were compared with a group of 98 with no history of affective disorder in a first-degree relative. Patients with a family history of affective disorder were more likely to have suffered from affective symptoms on follow-up. The conclusion was that "even when DSM III criteria are met hesitation is indicated in diagnosing schizophrenia in patients with a first degree relative with bipolar illness".

In the later paper, however, Kendler *et al* (1986) conclude that "The familial link between schizophrenia and at least a subgroup of schizoaffective disorders argues that the presence of prominent affective features, both depressive and manic, during the course of a chronic 'schizophrenic-like' illness need not indicate a familial predisposition to affective illness."

The question must be asked of the defenders of the Kraepelinian concept, where is the line to be drawn? Is it to be drawn so as to define schizophrenia restrictively, as Cloninger *et al* instruct us to do, and as it seems that Kendler in 1983 would have accepted, or is it to be drawn to include a substantial fraction of schizoaffective disorders, as Kendler *et al* in 1986 recommend. In this case we are faced with the problem of distinguishing the 'affective' types of schizoaffective disorder from the 'schizophrenic' types. But this is just what the investigations of Angst *et al* (1983) and Angst & Scharfetter (1990) and Gershon *et al* (1982, 1988) suggest cannot be achieved. The very existence of these illnesses is a challenge to the two-entities principle, as Kraepelin himself appreciated. Their genetic relationships as demonstrated by the recent studies deal a death-blow to the Kraepelinian system.

Winokur has wrestled long and hard with these problems (Winokur, 1984) and has been one of the stoutest defenders of the dichotomy. Even he, in collaboration with the Zurich group, has recognised the problems that the Kraepelinian system now faces. As a co-author (Stassen *et al*, 1988) reporting a study of 350 affected first-degree relatives of 269 in-patients with functional psychoses, he writes that "typical syndrome patterns clearly appeared in both populations [i.e. relatives and probands] . . . . Nevertheless our analyses revealed no clear breeding true of either affective disorders or schizophrenia."

Thus it is difficult to identify a coherent defence in the literature of the classic Kraepelinian position. It must be assumed that that position has given way to some form of the continuum hypothesis – either that there are a large number of different genetic entities, each with its own locus, that show substantial overlap in their phenotypic manifestations (Kendell, 1987), or that there are a number of different alleles at a single genetic locus (Crow, 1986*a*, 1987*a*). The first view has difficulty in explaining the extent and source of variation within families. The second faces the problem of the nature of the variation at the hypothetical locus. What sort of genes are these that show an apparently continuous variation? What sort of change in the gene could take place between different members of the same family?

The intergenerational change in the form of psychosis

One manifestation of within-family variation noted by a number of authors is an apparent increase in severity and change in form of psychosis between generations. One of the first to draw attention to this phenomenon was Rosenthal (1970). In a survey of risk of other psychiatric illness in first-degree relatives of patients with affective disorder, he noted an excess of schizophrenia in children (a mean of 2.3% in five studies), while the risk in parents and siblings remained within the 0.8% lifetime prevalence for the general population. Rosenthal asked, "From a genetic viewpoint why should schizophrenia have occurred at all in these families?"

Pollock & Malzberg (1940) collected family histories of psychosis over three generations and classified the probands as suffering from affective disorder or schizophrenia. In siblings, the ratio of schizophrenia to affective disorder was as predicted from the proband diagnosis (8 : 2 for schizophrenic probands, and 3 : 11 for affective), but for preceding generations the ratio was similar for the two groups of probands, 11 : 15 for schizophrenic and 3 : 7 for affective probands. Thus it appears that in preceding generations but not in siblings the rate of affective disorder is higher than would be predicted in relatives of patients with schizophrenia on a conventional view.

Slater (1953) reported similar findings. In his study of twins he recorded psychiatric illness in other relatives, and found the ratio of affective disorder to schizophrenia (4 : 3) to be particularly high in the parents of patients with schizophrenia. No excess of schizophrenia was found in the parents or siblings of patients with affective disorder. However, in an earlier study of manic–depressive illness, Slater (1936) reported:

> "a surprising feature had been the number of schizophrenics among the children. . . . In 10 of the 15 cases where manic–depressive subjects had been found by Dr Slater to have schizophrenic children he had been unable to find schizophrenia in other members of the patient's family or that of the husband or wife."

Two studies have examined parent–child pairs in which both members suffered from psychosis (Table. 3.2). Penrose (1968) identified 621 such

TABLE 3.2
Psychotic offspring of psychotic parents classified by diagnosis

Parents	Offspring	
	affective psychosis	*schizophrenia*
Penrose (1968)		
Affective psychosis	232	205
Schizophrenia	34	150
Powell et al *(1973)*		
Manic–depressive psychosis	10	15
Schizophrenia	0	9

pairs in a series of 5456 pairs of relatives with psychiatric disease admitted over a period of 18 years to the Ontario mental hospitals. Among the ill children of schizophrenic parents a diagnosis of schizophrenia preponderated over affective disorder in a ratio of almost 5 : 1. Among the in-patient children of affectively ill parents the ratio was only a little less than unity; schizophrenia was almost as common as affective disorder. In a similar study using the Aberdeen case register, Powell *et al* (1973) found schizophrenia in the children of schizophrenic parents, and affective illness among the children of parents with affective disorder, as expected. However, among the latter they found that for 10 cases of affective disorder, 15 cases of schizophrenia were also present.

The latest contribution to this literature is a study by Decina *et al* (1989) of a series of 24 parent–child pairs both admitted over a period of about 60 years to the same institution with diagnoses meeting DSM–III criteria for schizophrenia or affective disorder. While no case of affective disorder was found in the children of schizophrenic parents, 50% of children of parents with psychotic affective disorders presented with schizophrenia. The authors concluded that "The findings are consistent with the view that, in affected families, the severity of psychopathology increases from one generation to the next" and that "psychotic affective disorder in the parents may predispose to schizophrenia in the children."

Again the question must be asked – what sort of genes are these that change their phenotype so readily? What happens between generations in these cases? Do the genes reassort, recombine or even jump, or does their mode of expression change?

A related phenomenon in the case of both affective disorder and schizophrenia is the relative risk of psychosis in the different categories of first-degree relative (Table 3.3). The risk is greater in children than siblings, and greater in siblings than in parents. This is curious from a Mendelian point of view.

The phenomenon may be relevant to recent reports (for example from the NIMH Epidemiological Catchment Area Study; Klerman *et al*, 1985) of an apparent secular increase in affective disorder. These reports are generally based upon studies of affective disorder within families; again it may be that what we see is an increase in frequency or severity (or both) of illness between generations.

TABLE 3.3
Risk of illness in different categories of first-degree relative of probands with affective disorder and schizophrenia

	Bipolar affective disorder (Price et al, 1985)	Schizophrenia (Zerbin-Rudin, 1972)
Parents	4.8	6.3
Siblings	6.0	10.4
Children	9.5	13.7

From Crow (1986*b*).

Here we approach the central paradox of psychosis – why if these diseases are genetic in origin do they persist? Why are they so prevalent?

Book (1953) first suggested that schizophrenia was associated with a high rate of mutation, and was followed in this view by Lewis (1958) in his paper on fertility and mental illness. The suggestion may be relevant to affective disorders as well as to schizophrenia, and might relate also to intergenerational change. Perhaps what we see is a high rate of change at a particular locus that has the evolutionary advantage of generating new variants.

Where is the gene?

The *Lancet* (1987) discussed the alternative to Kraepelin's binary viewpoint – the continuum concept – emphasising what I accept is its corollary, that there should be a single genetic locus. Yet quite apart from the various claims to have established linkage for one or more of the psychoses that there have been, we have reasonable evidence that the affective disorders at least are sometimes sex-linked and sometimes not (Risch *et al*, 1986). Does this not indicate that heterogeneity is already established?

There remained one way in which homogeneity could yet be maintained – that the locus for psychosis should be within the pseudo-autosomal or exchange region of the sex chromosomes (Crow, 1987*b*, 1988), that small region of the short arms within which there is exchange of genetic material between X and Y chromosomes in male meiosis (Ferguson-Smith, 1965; Burgoyne, 1986). With such a locus there is the possibility of apparent sex linkage in a condition that generally follows an autosomal mode of inheritance.

There are other reasons for taking a sex-chromosomal locus for psychosis seriously. In a discussion of the excess of cases of sex-chromosome aneuploidy – particularly XXY and XXX – that has consistently been observed in populations of patients with psychosis, Forssman (1970) wrote:

> "Myself I am convinced that study of aberrations of the sex chromosomes will prove to have a radical effect on large sections of psychiatric thinking. . . . That several different types of gonosomal aberration are associated with an increased risk of functional psychosis is an observation which should make us stop and think."

A gene for psychosis on the sex chromosomes is widely discounted on the grounds of the autosomal pattern of transmission. A locus in the pseudo-autosomal region circumvents this problem.

The defining characteristic of pseudo-autosomal transmission is same-sex concordance – within families, individuals carrying a gene in this region will, above chance expectation, be of the same sex. This is so because when such a gene is inherited from a father it will be preferentially passed either on the X chromosome to daughters or on the Y chromosome to sons. By contrast, when the disease is inherited on an X chromosome from the mother it is equally likely to be passed to a daughter or a son.

Same-sex concordance in schizophrenia was first noted by Mott (1910), and was discussed in some detail by Penrose (1942) and Rosenthal (1962). The prediction that concordance by sex for psychosis will apply particularly to those cases in which inheritance is through the father has been tested in a series of 120 sibships that include at least two psychotic members (Crow *et al*, 1989). With paternal inheritance, pairs of siblings with schizophrenia were more likely to be of the same sex. Neither same-sex concordance itself nor its association with paternal transmission are dependent upon the excess of males that is present in this and some previous series (Crow *et al*, 1990).

The prediction of same-sex concordance in affective disorder can be tested in the existing literature for bipolar disorder (Table 3.4). There is an excess of same-sex over opposite-sex pairs and this cannot be accounted for by the excess of females that is also present.

The findings of the NIMH Collaborative Program on the Psychobiology of Depression with respect to familial transmission of bipolar illness (Rice *et al*, 1987) are also relevant. In this study of 187 families of bipolar patients, risk to relative was found to be unrelated to sex of proband or relative. However, there was heterogeneity in sex-specific sibling correlations, in that brother–sister correlations (0.36 for interview and 0.23 for history data) were significantly ($P < 0.05$ and $P < 0.005$ respectively) less than brother–brother (0.63 and 0.53) and sister–sister (0.53 and 0.54) correlations. The authors conclude that "the exact source of this heterogeneity is unclear . . . the mode of transmission appears to be complex and may suggest that the environmental similarity for siblings is sex specific". It could be that the correlation is genetic and that it reflects a locus in the pseudo-autosomal region.

TABLE 3.4

Distribution by sex in sibling pairs with bipolar affective illness

	Winokur et al (1969)[1]	Goetzl et al (1974)	Mendlewicz & Rainer (1974)[2]	Gershon et al (1982)[2]	Totals
Male–male	3	0	19	7	29
Male–female	4	0	19	15	38
Female–female	5	3	21	9	38
Same sex	67	Sign test (against 50 : 50 expectation) $z = 2.83$, $P < 0.0025$			
Opposite sex	38				

1. Data are as summarised by van Eerdewegh *et al* (1980).
2. Data are as abstracted by Risch *et al* (1986).

Conclusions

Contrary to established opinion, one is forced to conclude that little support for the Kraepelinian binary concept is to be found in genetic studies. Unquestionably there is a relationship between form of psychotic illness in a proband and form of illness in the first-degree relative, but there is also a lot of variation and, crucially, no lines of separation between the prototypical syndromes can be drawn on genetic grounds. Those studies that have included an unselected series of patients with psychotic illness as probands have failed to identify any natural line of cleavage that could serve to separate disorders that are predominantly affective from those that are primarily schizophrenic. Workers who claim that such a line can be drawn are not in agreement with each other, nor on occasion with themselves, as to where it should be drawn. It has to be concluded that there is a continuum of psychotic illness that includes variations within the affective (to include unipolar, bipolar and schizoaffective) and schizophrenic (to include variations in severity of defect symptoms) realms as well as between the major Kraepelinian prototypes.

Since this variation rests upon a genetic base it must be assumed that the psychosis gene either exists in different forms or is expressed in different ways. Further evidence for such genetic variation comes from studies that indicate that risk of a schizophrenic type of psychosis is increased in children of parents with affective illness. Already (to account for persistent high prevalence in the face of a fertility disadvantage) it has been proposed that the genes related to psychosis are subject to a high rate of mutation. Variation in form of illness within families and between generations further emphasises the possible role of mutation, epimutation (Holliday, 1987) or variations in mode of expression of the psychosis gene.

A locus for psychosis has been suggested in the pseudo-autosomal (exchange) region of the sex chromosomes. This could explain: (a) how X-linkage could appear in some families with affective disorder and autosomal transmission in others without any need to invoke heterogeneity; (b) the association between sex-chromosomal aneuploidies and psychosis; and (c) the phenomenon of concordance by sex for psychosis within families. Such concordance is found in family studies of both schizophrenic and affective illnesses.

References

AMERICAN PSYCHIATRIC ASSOCIATION (1980) *Diagnostic and Statistical Manual of Mental Disorders* (3rd edn) (DSM–III). Washington, DC: APA.

ANGST, J., FELDER, W. & LOHMEYER, B. (1979) Schizoaffective disorders: I, results of a genetic investigation. *Journal of Affective Disorders*, **1**, 139–153.

——, SCHARFETTER, C. & STASSEN, H. H. (1983) Classification of schizo-affective patients by multidimensional scaling and cluster analysis. *Psychiatria Clinica*, **16**, 254–264.

—— & —— (1985) Familial aspects of bipolar schizoaffective disorder, abstract S104. In *Affective Disorders, World Psychiatric Association Symposium, Athens, 1985*. WPA.

—— & —— (1990) Schizoaffective Psychosen. Ein Nosologischer Aergernis. In *Affektive Psychosen Kongress band DGPN* (eds E. Lungershausen, W. P. Kaschka & R. J. Witkowski). Stuttgart: Schattauer Verlag.

BECK, A. T. (1972) *Depression: Causes and Treatment*. Philadelphia: University of Pennsylvania Press.

BOOK, J. A. (1953) Schizophrenia as a gene mutation. *Acta Genetica et Statistica Medica*, **4**, 133–139.

BURGOYNE, P. S. (1986) Mammalian X and Y crossover. *Nature*, **319**, 258–259.

CLONINGER, C. R., MARTIN, R. L., GUZE, S. B., *et al* (1985) Diagnosis and prognosis in schizophrenia. *Archives of General Psychiatry*, **42**, 15–25.

CROW, T. J. (1986*a*) The continuum of psychosis and its implication for the structure of the gene. *British Journal of Psychiatry*, **149**, 419–429.

—— (1986*b*) Secular changes in affective disorder and variations in the psychosis gene. *Archives of General Psychiatry*, **43**, 1013–1014.

—— (1987*a*) Psychosis as a continuum and the virogene concept. *British Medical Bulletin*, **43**, 754–767.

—— (1987*b*) Pseudoautosomal locus for psychosis? *Lancet*, **ii**, 1532.

—— (1988) Sex chromosomes and psychosis: the case for a pseudoautosomal locus. *British Journal of Psychiatry*, **153**, 675–683.

——, DELISI, L. E. & JOHNSTONE, E. C. (1989) Concordance by sex in sibling pairs with schizophrenia is paternally inherited: evidence for a pseudoautosomal locus. *British Journal of Psychiatry*, **155**, 92–97.

——, —— & —— (1990) Reply. . . . A locus closer to the telomere? *British Journal of Psychiatry*, **156**, 416–420.

DECINA, P., LUSCAS, L. R., LINDER, J. R., *et al* (1989) Parent–child pairs with major psychiatric diseases, abstract 105. *142nd meeting of the American Psychiatric Association, San Francisco, May 1989*. Washington, DC: APA.

FERGUSON-SMITH, M. A. (1965) Karyotype-phenotype correlations in gonadal dysgenesis and their bearing on the pathogenesis of malformations. *Journal of Medical Genetics*, **2**, 142–155.

FLOR-HENRY, P. (1983) *Cerebral Basis of Psychopathology*. Bristol: Wright.

FORSSMAN, H. (1970) The mental implications of sex chromosome aberrations. *British Journal of Psychiatry*, **117**, 353–363.

GERSHON, E. S. & RIEDER, R. O. (1980) Are mania and schizophrenia genetically distinct? In *Mania, an Evolving Concept* (eds R. H. Belmaker & H. M. van Praag), pp. 97–109. New York: Spectrum.

——, HAMOVIT, J., GUROFF, J. J., *et al* (1982) A family study of schizo-affective, bipolar I, bipolar II, unipolar and normal control patients. *Archives of General Psychiatry*, **39**, 1157–1167.

——, DELISI, L. E., HAMOVIT, J., *et al* (1988) A controlled family study of chronic psychoses: schizophrenia and schizo-affective disorder. *Archives of General Psychiatry*, **45**, 328–336.

GOETZL, U., GREEN, R., WHYBROW, P., *et al* (1974) X linkage revisited; a further study of manic–depressive illness. *Archives of General Psychiatry*, **31**, 665–672.

HOLLIDAY, R. (1987) The inheritance of epigenetic defects. *Science*, **238**, 163–170.

KANT, O. (1942) The incidence of psychoses and other mental abnormalities in the families of recovered and deteriorated schizophrenic patients. *Psychiatric Quarterly*, **16**, 176–186.

KARLSSON, J. L. (1974) Inheritance of schizophrenia. *Acta Psychiatrica Scandinavica* (suppl. 274), 1–116.

KENDELL, R. E. (1987) Other functional psychoses. In *Companion to Psychiatric Studies* (4th edn) (eds R. E. Kendell & A. K. Zealley), pp. 363–377. Edinburgh: Churchill Livingstone.

—— & GOURLAY, J. (1970) The clinical distinction between the affective psychoses and schizophrenia. *British Journal of Psychiatry*, **117**, 261–266.

—— & BROCKINGTON, I. F. (1980) The identification of disease entities and the relationship between affective and schizophrenic psychoses. *British Journal of Psychiatry*, **137**, 324–331.

KENDLER, K. S. & HAYS, P. (1983) Schizophrenia subdivided by the family history of affective disorder. *Archives of General Psychiatry*, **40**, 951–955.
——, GRUENBERG, A. M. & TSUANG, M. T. (1986) A DSM–III family study of the nonschizophrenic psychotic disorders. *American Journal of Psychiatry*, **143**, 1098–1105.
KLERMAN, G. L., LAVORI, P. W., RICE, J., *et al* (1985) Birth-cohort trends in rates of major depressive disorder among relatives of patients with affective disorder. *Archives of General Psychiatry*, **42**, 689–693.
KRAEPELIN, E. (1920) Der Erscheinungsformen der Irreseins. *Zeitschrift fur Gesammte Neurologie u Psychiatrie*, **62**, 1–29. Trans. (1974) H. Marshall, Patterns of mental disorder. In *Themes and Variations in European Psychiatry* (eds S. R. Hirsch & M. Shepherd), pp. 9–30. Bristol: Wright.
LANCET (1987) A continuum of psychosis? *Lancet*, **ii**, 889–890.
LEWIS, A. J. (1958) Fertility and mental illness. *Eugenics Review*, **50**, 91–106.
LORANGER, A. W. (1981) Genetic independence of manic-depression and schizophrenia. *Acta Psychiatrica Scandinavica*, **63**, 444–452.
MAIER, W., HALLMAYER, J. & HEUN, R. (1989) A controlled family study in affective and schizophrenic disorders: support for continuum models and spectrum concepts. *1st World Congress of Psychiatric Genetics*, **1**, 35.
MENDLEWICZ, J. & RAINER, J. D. (1974) Morbidity risk and genetic transmission in manic depressive illness. *American Journal of Human Genetics*, **26**, 692–701.
MENNINGER, K., ELLENBERGER, H., PRUYSER, P., *et al* (1958) The unitary concept of mental illness. *Bulletin of the Menninger Clinic*, **22**, 4–12.
MOTT, F. W. (1910) Hereditary aspects of nervous and mental disease. *British Medical Journal*, **ii**, 1013–1020.
ØDEGÅRD, Ø. (1972) The multifactorial inheritance of predisposition to schizophrenia. In *Genetic Factors in "Schizophrenia"* (ed. A. R. Kaplan), pp. 256–275. Springfield: C. C. Thomas.
PENROSE, L. S. (1942) Auxiliary genes for determining sex as contributory causes of mental illness. *Journal of Mental Science*, **88**, 308–316.
—— (1968) Critical survey of schizophrenia genetics. In *Modern Perspectives in World Psychiatry* (ed. J. G. Howells), pp. 3–19. Edinburgh: Oliver & Boyd.
POLLOCK, H. M. & MALZBERG, B. (1940) Hereditary and environmental factors in the causation of manic–depressive psychosis and dementia praecox. *American Journal of Psychiatry*, **96**, 1227–1247.
POWELL, A., THOMSON, N., HALL, D. J., *et al* (1973) Parent–child concordance with respect to sex and diagnosis in schizophrenia and manic–depressive psychosis. *British Journal of Psychiatry*, **123**, 653–658.
PRICE, R. A., KIDD, K. K., PAULS, D. L. (1985) Multiple threshold models for affective disorders: the Yale–NIMH collaborative family study. *Journal of Psychiatric Research*, **19**, 553–546.
REICH, T., CLONINGER, C. R., SUAREZ, B., *et al* (1982) Genetics of the affective psychoses. In *Handbook of Psychiatry, vol. 3. Psychoses of Uncertain Aetiology* (eds L. Wing & J. K. Wing), pp. 147–159. Cambridge: Cambridge University Press.
RICE, J., REICH, T., ANDREASEN, N., *et al* (1987) The familial transmission of bipolar illness. *Archives of General Psychiatry*, **44**, 441–447.
RISCH, N., BARON, M. & MENDLEWICZ, J. (1986) Assessing the role of X-linked inheritance in bipolar-related major affective illness. *Journal of Psychiatric Research*, **20**, 275–288.
ROSENTHAL, D. (1962) Familial concordance by sex with respect to schizophrenia. *Psychological Bulletin*, **59**, 401–421.
—— (1970) *Genetic Theory and Abnormal Behavior*. New York: McGraw-Hill.
SLATER, E. T. O. (1936) Inheritance of manic–depressive insanity. *Lancet*, **i**, 429–431.
—— (1953) *Psychotic and Neurotic Illness in Twins*. London: HMSO.
SPITZER, R. L., ENDICOTT, J. R. & ROBINS, E. (1978) *Research Diagnostic Criteria (RDC) for a Selected Group of Functional Disorders* (3rd edn). New York: New York State Psychiatric Institute.
STASSEN, H. H., SCARFETTER, C., WINOKUR, G., *et al* (1988) Familial syndrome patterns in schizophrenia, schizoaffective disorder, mania, and depression. *European Archives of Psychiatry and Neurological Sciences*, **237**, 115–123.

WINOKUR, G. (1984) Psychosis in bipolar and unipolar affective illness with special reference to schizo-affective disorder. *British Journal of Psychiatry*, **145**, 236–242.

——— , CLAYTON, P. J. & REICH, T. (1969) *Manic–Depressive Illness*. St Louis: C. V. Mosby.

VAN EERDEWEGH, M. M., GERSHON, E. S. & VAN EERDEWEGH, P. M. (1980) X-chromosome threshold models of bipolar manic–depressive illness. *Journal of Psychiatric Research*, **15**, 215–238.

ZERBIN-RUDIN, E. (1972) Genetic research and the theory of schizophrenia. *International Journal of Mental Health*, **1**, 42–62.

4 The congenital and adult-onset psychoses: Kraepelin lost, Kraepelin found

ROBIN M. MURRAY and
EADBHARD O'CALLAGHAN

In an ideal world, the major psychoses would be subdivided according to the biological substrates underlying the different disorders. Since no such substrates had been demonstrated until very recently, most psychiatrists continue to rely upon Kraepelin's 'two-entity' theory in which schizophrenia is distinguished from manic–depression on the basis of phenomenology and outcome. Kraepelin's (1896) distinction of the two syndromes was heralded as a great advance in his day, as many medical disorders which had been initially described as syndromes had by then been shown each to have a distinct aetiology. Caution is, of course, required in extrapolating from syndrome to aetiology, as some syndromes can be produced by diverse causes (e.g. cardiac failure) while one cause can express itself in a variety of syndromes (e.g. syphilis). However, until recently it appeared that there was at least genetic validity in Kraepelin's distinction. This chapter re-examines the pillars supporting the Kraepelinian dichotomy; the conclusion is that in the light of our current knowledge, the psychoses can be more meaningfully divided into congenital and adult-onset types.

The present position

A phenomenological distinction?

Schizophrenia is a concept which has expanded and contracted over the decades, and whose borders and status remain much disputed (Foerster & Murray, 1987). There is little agreement about what constitutes the essential features. For example, Kraepelin pointed to a deterioration in the capacity to think as a primary characteristic, and Bleuler (1911) considered that if any clinical feature is pathognomonic of schizophrenia, it is a disturbance of thought. However, empirical research suggests that other psychotic patients demonstrate formal thought disorder at least as frequently as schizophrenic patients (Breakey & Goodell, 1972; Andreasen & Powers, 1974; Harrow *et al*, 1982; Grossman *et al*, 1986).

At one time, British psychiatrists thought that Schneider's first-rank symptoms represented the core of schizophrenia, and could be used to distinguish it from other psychotic disorders. It is now clear that this view was misplaced. Wing & Nixon (1975) noted that 13% of manic patients in the International Pilot Study of Schizophrenia exhibited first-rank symptoms, while Carpenter *et al* (1973) reported their presence in 23% of patients with a diagnosis of affective disorder. Furthermore, almost a third of schizophrenics do not exhibit first-rank symptoms at all (Mellor, 1970; Koehler, 1979), and, in any case, their presence has no predictive value (Brockington *et al*, 1978).

As discussed in Chapter 1, Kendell and colleagues (Kendell & Gourlay, 1970; Kendell & Brockington, 1980) have shown that, even using the most sophisticated statistical techniques to try to separate the manifestations of schizophrenia from those of manic–depression, no point of rarity can be found. Thus, we cannot rely on clinical phenomena alone to distinguish between schizophrenia and manic–depression, and Kraepelin's first principle is seen to be false. One must, however, enter a caveat here. Cloninger *et al* (1985) have been able to demonstrate a 'point of rarity' of symptoms between schizophrenia and other psychiatric disorders. Schizophrenia, as defined by these authors' scale, was familial and had a poor outcome, leading the authors to claim that they had validated the disease concept. However, this claim has been ridiculed by some (Grayson, 1986), and dismissed by others, on the grounds that the definition was so narrow that it did not resemble the normal concept of schizophrenia. However, this may be an inappropriate basis on which to reject the findings, as discussed below.

An inevitable deterioration?

Current operational diagnostic criteria for schizophrenia have been narrowed so that they may better predict a course of illness typical of that described by Kraepelin, with progressive deterioration (Foerster & Murray, 1987). In his ten-year follow-up study of 1054 unspecified admissions, Kraepelin (1913) described a poor outcome for 83% of the sample; only 4% of the patients had been discharged well and not readmitted subsequently. However, his study was retrospective, and therefore biased towards poor-outcome cases. Samples consisting of first-admission schizophrenics are more representative of persons experiencing the illness, and cast doubt upon Kraepelin's pessimistic view of outcome. For instance, his view was challenged by Mayer-Gross's (1932) 16-year follow-up study which reported that 35% of patients had made a "social recovery". More recently, Bleuler (1978), from the perspective of a 23-year follow-up, suggested that after five

TABLE 4.1
Long-term outcome studies of schizophrenia

	No. of subjects	Years to follow-up	Type	Outcome (%)		
				good[1]	intermediate	poor[2]
Kraepelin (1913)	1054	10	Retrospective	4	12	83
Brown *et al* (1966)	111	5	Retrospective	35	37	28
Bleuler (1972)	208	23	Prospective	30	34	35
Ciompi (1980)	282	37	Retrospective	36	40	23
Huber *et al* (1980)	502	22	Prospective	22	40	35
Harding *et al* (1987)	253	20	Prospective	26	37	38

1. Functioning adequately in all areas of life without evidence of psychosis.
2. Poor functioning/prolonged hospital stay/suicide.

years schizophrenia does not progress further; indeed, he believed there may be improvement not only in symptoms but also in work and social adjustment. As can be seen from Table 4.1, the majority of modern prospective studies confirm the view that schizophrenia does not invariably result in progressive deterioration. When viewed collectively, these studies suggest that the outcome in schizophrenia is not at all as bleak as was suggested by Kraepelin.

Examining the other side of the coin, it is by no means clear that patients with affective disorder have an invariably good prognosis. Current estimates indicate that as many as a third of bipolar patients have a poor social outcome (Clayton, 1981). Additionally, Lee & Murray (1988), who carried out an 18-year follow-up of a series of 89 depressed patients admitted to the Maudsley Hospital, reported that less than a fifth of the series had remained entirely well, whereas 41% of first-admission cases had "very poor outcome"; 13% of the series had subsequent episodes of schizoaffective disorder, and 7% developed either chronic paranoid or schizophrenic psychosis. Akiskal (1982) reported that 26% of patients with primary depressive illness became social "invalids", and similarly Paykel & Weissman (1973) reported that poor social outcome was not uncommon. This leads to the conclusion that outcome in affective disorder is considerably worse than Kraepelin originally envisaged.

A comparison, therefore, of outcome studies of schizophrenia and affective disorder calls into question the second of the principles upon which Kraepelin based his differentiation between the two syndromes. Furthermore, there is considerable variation in outcome among patients given a diagnosis of schizophrenia. A minority do indeed have the poor prognosis originally described by Kraepelin, but others do well, not only in having few if any readmissions to hospital, but also in terms of work and social functioning.

Genetic validity?

Kraepelin (1896) was aware of the relevance of familial factors to the aetiology of dementia praecox. Since then many studies have confirmed that the disorder is indeed familial (Murray *et al*, 1986; McGuffin *et al*, 1987), one of the most rigorous of these being that of Kendler *et al* (1985). However, the latter authors also reported that bipolar disorder occurred twice as frequently among the relatives of schizophrenics as among the relatives of a control group.

Furthermore, the examination of families multiply affected by psychotic disorder has revealed a number of large pedigrees containing some individuals affected by schizophrenia and others by bipolar affective disorder (Waddington & Youssef, 1988; St Clair *et al*, 1989). The recent literature has also shown diagnostic overlap in twin and triplet studies. For example, McGuffin *et al* (1982), who applied standardised interviews and blind rating to a set of monozygotic triplets, noted that two had a diagnosis of schizophrenia and the third affective psychosis. (Our recent perusal of records of the course of these triplets over the subsequent eight years has shown their illness to have become more alike than was initially reported.) Dalby *et al* (1986) reported a similar finding. McGuffin *et al* (1984, 1987) also reviewed the monozygotic twins originally described by Gottesman & Shields (1972), and noted the occurrence of five pairs in which the proband was diagnosed as schizophrenic according to DSM–III, yet the second twin received a diagnosis of affective disorder according to DSM–III (American Psychiatric Association, 1980).

The situation is further complicated by claims (Crow, 1986) of an increased morbid risk of schizophrenia among the relatives of patients with affective psychosis. However, the studies quoted by Crow are dated and therefore subject to diagnostic artefact, as operational criteria were not generally employed. In a recent study of a consecutive series of 73 psychotics which used such criteria, Foerster *et al* (1991*a*) showed that the morbid risk of DSM–III schizophrenia was increased only in the first-degree relatives of DSM–III schizophrenics and not in the relatives of affective psychotics. The morbid risk of affective disorder was higher, but not significantly so, in the relatives of affective psychotic probands compared with the relatives of schizophrenic probands.

Crow (1986) quotes data from Ødegård (1972) as supporting a genetic continuum. However, a more careful examination of Ødegård's results shows that it was those schizophrenic probands "without registered defect" (schizoaffective and allied conditions) whose relatives had an increased risk of affective psychosis; relatives of schizophrenic probands "with severe defect" had much lower risks of affective psychosis and higher risks of schizophrenia. These data are consonant with many other studies. For example, McCabe *et al* (1971) reported a morbid risk for affective disorder of 10.0% in the first-degree relatives of probands with "good prognosis schizophrenia" but only 1.5% in the relatives of probands with "poor prognosis schizophrenia". The pattern of morbid risk for schizophrenia was reversed, being 3.6% and 11.6% in the relatives of "good" and "poor prognosis" probands respectively. Pope & Lipinsky (1978), who reviewed this field, concluded that "schizophrenics of the good prognosis categories show typically two to three times as much familial affective illness as schizophrenia; poor prognosis groups show a two to threefold difference in the opposite direction".

Support for the idea that acute schizoaffective disorder is more closely related genetically to affective disorder than is classic schizophrenia comes from Murray *et al* (1984). This study concerned all those monozygotic twins who had presented to the Maudsley Hospital between 1948 and 1982 and received a clinical diagnosis of schizophrenia or possible schizophrenia; there were 68 such twins but 6 were discarded because of insufficient information on the cotwins. The Research Diagnostic Criteria (RDC; Spitzer *et al*, 1978) were then applied to all the carefully collected clinical information on both the proband and cotwin in the remaining 62 pairs. Twenty-four probands met the RDC for schizophrenia and 19 the RDC for schizoaffective disorder. Only 5 cotwins (21%) of the 24 probands with RDC schizophrenia received no psychiatric diagnosis. Eight of the cotwins met the RDC for schizophrenia, while 5 met the DSM–III criteria for schizotypal personality disorder. Only two cotwins met the RDC for schizoaffective disorder and one for major affective disorder. The remainder were psychiatrically well.

Among the cotwins of the 19 probands with RDC schizoaffective disorder, only a minority (two) again escaped any psychiatric diagnosis. But there was a marked difference in the diagnoses attributed to the ill cotwins. Only one was diagnosed as schizophrenic and one as DSM–III schizotypal personality, while six received a diagnosis of RDC schizoaffective disorder and six of major affective disorder.

Thus, cotwins of schizoaffective probands tended to be diagnosed as either suffering from schizoaffective disorder or major affective disorder (64%) but only rarely as schizophrenic or schizotypal (10%). On the other hand, the cotwins of schizophrenic probands were more frequently diagnosed as schizophrenic or schizotypal (54%) than as having schizoaffective or major affective disorders (12%).

The obvious implication is that RDC schizoaffective disorder is genetically relatively distinct from RDC schizophrenia and that the latter is more closely related genetically to schizotypal personality disorder than to affective disorder. Support for the relationship between schizoaffective disorder and affective disorder comes from an earlier twin study by Cohen *et al* (1972) who, without benefit of operational definitions, showed that the monozygotic concordance rate for schizoaffective disorder (50%) was more than twice that for schizophrenia (23.5%) but not statistically significantly higher than for manic–depression (38.5%). Much evidence does suggest that acute schizoaffective disorder is the most familial of the functional psychoses in the sense of having the highest risks of psychosis to relatives (Scharrfetter & Nusperli, 1980; Gershon *et al*, 1982, 1988).

Support for the relationship between narrowly defined schizophrenia and schizotypal disorder comes from six studies which have shown increased rates of schizotypal personality disorder in the relatives of RDC schizophrenics (Kendler, 1988). Furthermore, Kety *et al* (1978) found rates of schizotypal personality disorder in the relatives of adoptees with acute schizophrenia which were substantially lower than the rates in the relatives of adoptees with chronic schizophrenia. In their reanalysis using DSM–III criteria, Kendler & Gruenberg (1984) found schizotypal personality disorder no more common in the biological relatives of adoptees with atypical or schizophreniform disorders than in the relatives of control adoptees.

In view of these data, our Maudsley twin probands were split into those who met Kety's criteria for acute and for chronic schizophrenia; none of the 12 probands who met the acute criteria had a chronic schizophrenic cotwin, though 3 (25%) had an acute schizophrenic cotwin. Among the 23 cotwins of chronic probands, 8 (35%) received a diagnosis of chronic schizophrenia, while 4 (17%) received a diagnosis of acute schizophrenia.

All of the above studies are consistent with the notion that the appropriate genetic distinction is not between schizophrenia and affective psychosis but rather between acute schizophrenia, schizoaffective disorder, and affective psychosis on the one hand, and chronic schizophrenia and schizotypal personality on the other. As Kety (1980) states "The group of acute functional psychoses differs so much from classical schizophrenia that it is difficult to see what advantage inheres in our continuing to confound them".

Summary of the present position

Thus, the distinction between manic–depression and schizophrenia in terms of phenomenology, outcome, and familial homotypy is essentially flawed. Crow (1986; see also Chapter 3) has interpreted these data as indicating that there is no true distinction between the psychoses; rather they lie along a genetic continuum which starts with unipolar depression at one end, and moves through bipolar affective disorder and schizoaffective disorder, to chronic schizophrenia at the other, most 'genetic', pole of the continuum. However, this view has little explanatory power, and ignores the evidence that the relatives of chronic schizophrenics are at less risk of affective psychosis than the relatives of schizoaffective and bipolar probands.

A more plausible view is that the reason for the failure to establish a valid subdivision of the psychoses is not because they are a single disorder as Crow hypothesises, but rather because the distinction has been made at the wrong point. The evidence we have reviewed from phenomenological, outcome and genetic studies suggests that Kraepelin's original concept of dementia praecox represents a much more distinct entity than the modern notion of schizophrenia. Unfortunately, dementia praecox has been subsumed in a wider range of disorders which resemble it in featuring positive symptoms, but differ markedly in aetiology, epidemiology and brain morphology. Our contention is that not only was Bleuler's (1911) concept of schizophrenia too broad, but that in his later years Kraepelin himself became overinclusive in his definition of the disorder.

Neurodevelopmental deviance in schizophrenia

Structural brain abnormality

Kraepelin was convinced that dementia praecox had a structural correlate in the brain, but it is only in the last decade that firm evidence has been produced to support this. Neuropathological studies (Bogerts *et al*, 1985; Brown *et al*, 1986; Jakob & Beckmann, 1986) show smaller temporal lobe structures in the brains of schizophrenics and, in most cases, an absence of gliosis. Together these suggest developmental rather than degenerative pathology (Roberts *et al*, 1987). Recently, Bogerts *et al* (1990) confirmed that up to 40% of post-mortem schizophrenic brains show failure of migration of pre-alpha cells in the entorhinal cortex. This suggests that some schizophrenias are a consequence of neurodevelopmental disorder, since the migration of these cells is largely complete by the neonatal period.

Neuropathological studies have, by necessity, been carried out on samples too small, and patients too poorly documented, to correlate clinical findings with the structural changes. However, neuroimaging studies have taken this process further. Thus, it has been demonstrated that the cerebral ventricular enlargement found in a proportion of schizophrenic patients is not the result of treatment (Johnstone *et al*, 1976; Williams *et al*, 1985), and is present at the onset of the illness (Nyback *et al*, 1982; Weinberger *et al*, 1982). Indeed it is associated with poor pre-morbid adjustment (Weinberger *et al*, 1980; DeLisi *et al* 1983; Williams *et al*, 1985) and in some studies with a history of obstetric complications (Murray *et al*, 1988; Lewis *et al*, 1989).

Since only a subset of schizophrenic patients demonstrate these changes, investigators have attempted to find the clinical parameters of this subpopulation. One of the most consistent findings is that of cognitive impairment (Johnstone *et al*, 1976) but significant relationships have also been reported with more negative symptoms (Andreasen *et al*, 1982; Pearlson *et al*, 1984*a*), a poorer response to neuroleptics (Luchins *et al*, 1984), and poor outcome (Williams *et al*, 1985). An interesting finding is that males are more likely to exhibit structural brain abnormalities on computerised tomography (CT) or magnetic resonance imaging (MRI) scan than females. Castle & Murray (1991) reviewed ten studies (6 CT and 4 MRI) which report more morphological abnormalities among males than females. Bogerts *et al* (1990) also found that the brains of male schizophrenic patients showed more neuropathological abnormalities than their female counterparts.

Thus, there appears to be a subgroup of schizophrenic patients who demonstrate morphological brain changes which antedate the development of the positive clinical syndrome. The neuropathological and CT findings are supported by recent MRI reports of reduced volume of temporal lobe grey matter (Suddath *et al*, 1989). These brain changes appear to signify some early developmental deviance and occur most commonly among male patients and among those with poor pre-morbid adjustment, evidence of cognitive impairment, and a poor outcome.

Early development

Of the environmental factors that have been associated with schizophrenia, the most consistently reported are obstetric complications (OCs). Here the term is used in the broad sense to define deviations from the normal course of events during pregnancy, birth and early neonatal life. The obstetric histories of schizophrenic patients are characterised by an excess of complications when compared with controls (McNeil, 1987) and to patients suffering from other psychiatric disorders (McNeil & Kaij, 1978; Lewis & Murray, 1987). Furthermore, those patients with a history of OCs develop the disorder on average five years before those without such a history, and male schizophrenics have an excess of OCs when compared with females (Wilcox & Nasrallah, 1987; Pearlson *et al*, 1989; Foerster *et al*, 1991*a*).

Murray *et al* (1985) suggested that OCs may be one of several environmental factors which may act independently to predispose individuals without any obvious genetic predisposition to the subsequent development of schizophrenia. An alternative view is that OCs may be an indirect indicator of some earlier insult to the nervous system, or a secondary consequence of some genetic defect in neural development (Owen *et al*, 1988; Goodman, 1988).

The excess of minor physical anomalies (MPAs) in schizophrenics provides a further indication of developmental disruption. These trivial abnormalities in ectodermal development are of little consequence in themselves, but ectodermal development during foetal life closely parallels that of the central nervous system, and MPAs are known to occur in excess in patients with developmental disorders (Smith, 1976). Relatively few studies have examined schizophrenic patients for such abnormalities, but all of those which have (Gualtieri *et al*, 1982; Guy *et al*, 1983; Green *et al*, 1987) report increased MPAs among schizophrenic patients compared with controls. Green *et al* (1989) noted that MPAs predict a younger age of onset of schizophrenia while Waddington *et al* (1990) reported that MPAs are more common among male patients and among those who are cognitively impaired.

Thus OCs and MPAs both occur in excess among persons with schizophrenia, both appear more commonly among males, and both predict an early onset of the disorder. Finally, both implicate a pathological process operating early in life when the nervous system is at its most vulnerable.

Kraepelin had little doubt that some individuals with dementia praecox had behaved differently, even as children, from their siblings and peers. These abnormalities were encapsulated by Kretschmer (1921) as 'schizoid personality', which he described as characterised by eccentricity, solitariness and an aloof manner. In a recent controlled study in which the mothers of 73 DSM–III-diagnosed psychotics were interviewed, Foerster *et al* (1991*a*,*b*) confirmed pre-morbid schizoid and schizotypal traits and poor social adjustment in the childhoods of a proportion of the schizophrenics. Furthermore, those schizophrenics who were abnormal as children had an early onset of psychosis and were characterised by a family history of schizophrenia or a history of OCs or low birth weight. Interestingly, the study revealed that pre-morbid deficits and schizoid/schizotypal personality traits were largely confined to those males who subsequently developed schizophrenia.

Do acute psychotics have evidence of neurodevelopmental abnormality?

Acute affective psychosis

Now that it is clear that a proportion of patients with schizophrenia have evidence of neurodevelopmental impairment, it is incumbent upon us to ascertain whether the same holds for affective psychosis. To our knowledge there have not been systematic studies of MPAs in patients with primary affective disorder. Similarly, there have been few studies of OCs or of pre-morbid personality in such patients. However, Foerster *et al* (1991*a*,*b*) addressed both these issues. A developmental history was obtained from patients' mothers with the interviewer 'blind' to whether the patient was suffering from schizophrenia or affective psychosis. Mothers gave evidence of OCs for 40% of probands with schizophrenia but for only 7% of probands with affective psychosis. As noted previously, poor social adjustment and schizoid and schizotypal traits in childhood were common among male pre-schizophrenics. However, they were rare among those who developed affective psychosis. Similarly, soft neurological signs and cognitive defects are uncommon in patients with primary affective disorder (Woods *et al*, 1986).

What of those other findings which have been associated with neurodevelopmental abnormality in schizophrenia? Unfortunately, neuropathological studies of patients with affective psychosis are relatively scarce. Jeste *et al* (1988) discovered 15 such reports but the majority of these only included patients with affective disorders as controls for comparison with schizophrenics. Furthermore, 14 of these 15 studies had sample sizes smaller than 18 patients. The only substantial study is that of Brown *et al* (1986), who compared the brains of 26 schizophrenic patients with those of 41 unipolar depressives and 29 bipolar patients. The schizophrenics had larger cerebral ventricles, their brains were 6% lighter, and they had thinner parahippocampal cortices than the patients with affective disorder. The schizophrenics showed dilatation of the temporal horn of the lateral ventricle but no such change was noted among the patients with affective disorder.

A number of CT and MRI studies have been carried out in patients with affective psychosis but many of these have been concerned with elderly (Jacoby & Levy, 1980), severe, or resistant (Standish-Barry *et al*, 1982) forms of the disorder (Targum *et al*, 1983; Luchins *et al*, 1984; Pearlson *et al*, 1984*a,b*; Shima *et al*, 1984; Dolan *et al*, 1985; Roy-Byrne *et al*, 1988). Those studies of more representative samples show that structural abnormality is less common in affective disorder than in schizophrenia. For example, Shettar *et al* (1990) found no difference in temporal and hippocampal volume between depressed patients and controls in contrast to the findings of Suddath *et al* (1989), who reported that schizophrenics have decreased temporal volume when compared with controls. Similarly, Johnstone *et al* (1989) reported that while temporal lobe structures of manic–depressives, as determined by MRI, did not differ from controls, schizophrenic patients differed significantly from both controls and manic–depressives. Interestingly, among the schizophrenics, only males showed evidence of enlarged temporal horns.

Thus, structural abnormalities appear less common in affective psychosis than in schizophrenia. Furthermore, when they do occur they appear to be associated with late rather than early onset. Indeed, Sacchetti *et al* (1987) suggest that when ventricular enlargement occurs in affective disorder, it does so in late-onset cases in which the affective disorder itself may be a manifestation of some primary brain disorder such as cerebral vascular disease.

Acute schizophrenia

Thus, affective psychosis differs from early-onset, poor-outcome schizophrenia in that the latter but not the former shows evidence of neurodevelopmental abnormality. But what about that third group variously described as suffering from schizoaffective disorder, or acute or good-prognosis schizophrenia?

In terms of clinical manifestations (abrupt onset, positive symptoms, good response to neuroleptics and good outcome) these patients share many characteristics with affective psychotics. Such patients are also similar to affective psychotics in having an unremarkable pre-morbid personality and in rarely having a history of OCs (McNeil & Kaij, 1978; Foerster *et al*, 1991*a,b*). Good-outcome schizophrenics do however show cognitive impairment. For example, Lindenmeyer *et al* (1989) showed that a group of 35 RDC schizoaffective patients showed significantly less cognitive abnormality than a comparison group of 35 RDC schizophrenics, matched for age and duration of illness.

We noted earlier that the rates of schizoaffective and affective disorder in the relatives of good-outcome schizophrenics are high while rates of schizophrenia and schizotypal personality disorder are low. Schizophrenics with a relative suffering from bipolar affective illness are especially likely to show affective symptoms during their acute illness, and to have few residual symptoms in remission (Kendler & Hays, 1983). Furthermore, Owen *et al* (1988) have shown using CT that schizophrenics with a family history of affective disorder are less likely to have enlarged cerebral ventricles than other schizophrenics. CT studies also suggest that good-outcome schizophrenics are less likely to have ventricular enlargement than chronic schizophrenics (Kolakowska *et al*, 1985).

Neuropathological investigations have generally been carried out on that segment of the schizophrenic population whose brains are available on death. Consequently, the sample is heavily skewed towards chronic patients residing in mental hospitals, and few acute schizophrenics have been studied.

Another important factor that distinguishes good-outcome from poor-outcome schizophrenia is gender. Female schizophrenics have a far more favourable outcome than males. This appears to have been true even in the pre-neuroleptic era, as Kraepelin himself commented on it. Females have more affective and atypical symptoms while males more frequently exhibit the classic symptoms of schizophrenia (Lewine, 1981; Goldstein & Link, 1988; Castle & Murray, 1991). Males, as noted earlier, show more structural abnormalities in the brain as well as more neurological abnormalities (Marcus *et al*, 1985; Woods *et al*, 1987), more MPAs (Waddington *et al*, 1990) and more OCs. Males tend to show a younger age of onset of schizophrenia than females (Lewine, 1988; Angermeyer & Kuhn, 1988); this is not a consequence of the manner in which age of onset is defined (Loranger, 1984; Hafner *et al*, 1989).

These data strongly suggest that acute, good-outcome schizophrenia is not consequent upon neurodevelopmental disorder, and that the sex differences in schizophrenia reflect the fact that a lower proportion of female than male patients who present with schizophrenic symptoms have the neurodevelopmental, early-onset and poor-outcome type (Castle & Murray, 1991).

Classifying schizophrenia into congenital and adult-onset type

It will be evident that there is a common theme running through the discussion hitherto: the classification of the functional psychoses should be based on a developmental principle. Such a classification, we believe, would go some way towards explaining the phenotypic differences in the psychoses, and would subdivide schizophrenia into two main groups whose prototypic characteristics are summarised in Table 4.2.

Congenital schizophrenia

This term by definition implies that abnormality is present (although not necessarily recognisable) at birth. We postulate that this type may arise as a consequence of a genetic defect in the control of neuronal proliferation and migration. This results in smaller temporal lobe structures as visualised by neuroimaging studies, and post-mortem evidence of migration failure of the pre-alpha cells in the entorhinal cortex (Jones & Murray, 1991). Schizotypal personality may represent a partial expression of the responsible gene(s). A similar clinical and neuropathological picture may also result from early environmental insult in foetal or neonatal life. These persons are more likely to show evidence of early developmental anomalies (OCs and MPAs), and to have shown schizoid pre-morbid personality traits or social impairment as early as primary-school years. Such individuals present to

TABLE 4.2
Prototypic characteristics of the different schizophrenias

	Congenital type	*Adult-onset type*
Clinical characteristics	Insidious onset Marked negative symptoms Cognitive impairment Few affective symptoms	Acute onset Mainly positive symptoms No cognitive impairment Excess of affective symptoms
Outcome	Poor response to neuroleptics Poor prognosis	Good response to neuroleptics Good prognosis
Epidemiology	Early onset of psychosis (<20 years) Male excess No increase in recent life events	Onset throughout life Female excess Increase in recent life events

Morbid risk in relatives	Increased risk of schizophrenia
	  and schizotypal disorders
		Increased risk of schizoaffective
		  and affective disorders

Developmental abnormality	Winter birth excess Excess of obstetric complications Excess of minor physical anomalies Presence of neurological soft signs Poor pre-morbid functioning	Normal birth distribution No excess of obstetric complications No excess of minor physical anomalies No neurological soft signs Normal pre-morbid functioning

Structural changes	Ventricular enlargement on CT
	Temporal lobe volume decreased
	  on MRI
	Heterotropic pre-alpha cells at
	  post-mortem
		No primary structural abnormalities

the psychiatric services earlier, exhibit more negative symptoms, and show morphological brain changes and cognitive impairment. In their clinical presentation, age of onset and male predominance, this group reflects the original description of dementia praecox by Kraepelin.

Adult-onset schizophrenia

Our contention is that all other patients who exhibit the positive symptoms of schizophrenia, and are currently classified under the category of schizophrenia, are in fact not suffering from dementia praecox. Such patients have little in common aetiologically with cases of dementia praecox, lack the developmental attributes of the congenital forms of schizophrenia, and share many features with other adult-onset functional psychoses at present classified outside the schizophrenia syndrome. The most numerous patients within the group of adult-onset schizophrenias are those patients who have a disorder which is genetically related to affective disorder. In essence, we consider that there exists an adult-onset psychotic disorder, under a high degree of genetic control, in which the phenotypic expression of the mutant genes ranges from classic manic–depression through schizoaffective disorder to acute schizophrenia.

The adult-onset schizophrenias also include other conditions of lesser importance which share a common symptom pathway. These comprise the paranoid psychoses, the so-called late paraphrenias, and those schizophrenias consequent upon drug and alcohol abuse.

Conclusion

The pillars supporting the Kraepelin dichotomy of the functional psychoses are crumbling. There are two main interpretations of the relevant data. The first is that schizophrenia and manic–depression are a single disorder lying along a continuum with a single aetiology (Crow, 1986). Our interpretation is diametrically opposed to such a view. We contend that several genetic and environmental aetiologies underlie the functional psychoses, but that there is a single group (the congenital psychoses) which can be distinguished from other forms whose manifestations are confined to adult life. Thus, while we find no support for the current 'Kraepelinian' distinction between manic–depression and schizophrenia ('Kraepelin lost'), we believe that the congenital psychoses closely resemble Kraepelin's original description of dementia praecox ('Kraepelin found').

References

AKISKAL, H. S. (1982) Factors associated with incomplete recovery in primary depressive illness. *Journal of Clinical Psychiatry*, **43**, 266–271.

AMERICAN PSYCHIATRIC ASSOCIATION (1980) *Diagnostic and Statistical Manual of Mental Disorders* (3rd edn) (DSM–III). Washington, DC: APA.

ANDREASEN, N. C. & POWERS, P. S. (1974) Overinclusive thinking in mania and schizophrenia. *British Journal of Psychiatry*, **125**, 452–456.

——, OLSEN, S. A., DENNERT, J. W., *et al* (1982) Ventricular enlargement in schizophrenia: relationship to positive and negative symptoms. *American Journal of Psychiatry*, **139**, 297–302.

ANGERMEYER, M. C. & KUHN, L. (1988) Gender differences in schizophrenia: an overview. *European Archives of Psychiatry and Neurological Sciences*, **237**, 351–364.

BLEULER, E. (1911) *Dementia Praecox or the Group of Schizophrenias* (trans. J. Zinkin, 1950). New York: International Universities Press.

BLEULER, M. (1972) *Die schizophrenen Geistesstorungen im Lichte langjahriger Kranken-und Familiengeschichten.* Stuttgart: George Thieme, Verlag.

—— (1978) *The Schizophrenic Disorders; The Long Term Patient and Family Studies* (trans. S. M. Clemens). New Haven: Yale University Press.

BOGERTS, B., MEERTZ, E. & SCHONFELDT-BAUSCH, R. (1985) Basal ganglia and limbic system pathology in schizophrenia. *Archives of General Psychiatry*, **42**, 784–791.

——, ASHTARI, M., DEGREEF, G. M., *et al* (1990) Reduced temporal limbic structure volumes on magnetic resonance images in first episode schizophrenia. *Psychiatry Research: Neuroimaging*, **35**, 1–13.

BREAKEY, W. R. & GOODELL, H. (1972) Thought disorder in mania and schizophrenia evaluated by Bannister's grid test for schizophrenic thought disorder. *British Journal of Psychiatry*, **120**, 391–395.

BROCKINGTON, I. F., KENDELL, R. E. & LEFF, J. P. (1978) Definitions of schizophrenia: concordance and prediction of outcome. *Psychological Medicine*, **8**, 387–398.

BROWN, R., COLTER, N., CORSELLIS, J. A. N., *et al* (1986) Postmortem evidence of structural brain changes in schizophrenia: differences in brain weight, temporal horn area and parahippocampal gyrus compared with affective disorder. *Archives of General Psychiatry*, **43**, 36–42.

CARPENTER, W. T., STRAUSS, J. S. & MULEH, S. (1973) Are there pathognomonic symptoms of schizophrenia? *Archives of General Psychiatry*, **28**, 847–852.

CASTLE, D. J. & MURRAY, R. M. (1991) The neurodevelopmental basis of sex differences in schizophrenia. *Psychological Medicine* (in press).

CIOMPI, L. (1980) The natural history of schizophrenia in the long term. *British Journal of Psychiatry*, **136**, 413–420.

CLAYTON, P. J. (1981) The epidemiology of bipolar affective disorder. *Comprehensive Psychiatry*, **22**, 31–43.

CLONINGER, C. R., MARTIN, R. L., GUZE, S. B., *et al* (1985) Diagnosis and prognosis in schizophrenia. *Archives of General Psychiatry*, **42**, 15–25.

COHEN, S. M., ALLEN, M. G., POLLIN, W., *et al* (1972) Relationship of schizoaffective psychosis to manic depressive psychosis and schizophrenia. *Archives of General Psychiatry*, **26**, 539–546.

CROW, T. J. (1986) The continuum of psychosis and its implication for the structure of the gene. *British Journal of Psychiatry*, **149**, 419–429.

DALBY, J. T., MORGAN, D. & LEE, M. L. (1986) Schizophrenia and mania in identical twin brothers. *Journal of Nervous and Mental Disease*, **174**, 304–308.

DELISI, L. E., SCHWARTZ, C. C., TARGUM, S. D., *et al* (1983) Ventricular brain enlargement and outcome of acute schizophreniform disorder. *Psychiatry Research*, **9**, 169–171.

DOLAN, R. J., CALLOWAY, S. P. & MANN, A. H. (1985) Cerebral ventricular size in depressed subjects. *Psychological Medicine*, **15**, 873–878.

FOERSTER, A. & MURRAY, R. M. (1987) Schizophrenia: is the concept disintegrating? *Journal of Psychopharmacology*, **1**, 133–139.

——, LEWIS, S. E., OWEN, M. J., *et al* (1991a) Do risk factors for schizophrenia also predict poor premorbid functioning in psychosis? *Schizophrenia Research* (in press).

——, ——, ——, *et al* (1991b) Premorbid personality in psychosis: effects of sex and diagnosis. *British Journal of Psychiatry*, **158**, 171–176.

GERSHON, E. S., HAMOVIT, J., GUROFF, J. J., *et al* (1982) A family study of schizoaffective bipolar I, bipolar II, unipolar and normal control probands. *Archives of General Psychiatry*, **39**, 1157–1167.

———, DeLISI, L. E., HAMOVIT, J., *et al* (1988) A controlled family study of chronic psychoses, schizophrenia and schizoaffective disorder. *Archives of General Psychiatry*, **45**, 328–336.

GOLDSTEIN, J. M. & LINK, B. G. (1988) Gender differences in the clinical expression of schizophrenia. *Journal of Psychiatric Research*, **22**, 141–155.

GOODMAN, R. (1988) Are complications of pregnancy and birth causes of schizophrenia? *Developmental Medicine and Child Neurology*, **30**, 391–400.

GOTTESMAN, I. I. & SHIELDS, J. (1972) *Schizophrenia and Genetics: A Twin Study Vantage Point.* London: Academic Press.

GRAYSON, D. (1986) Asessment of evidence for a categorical view of schizophrenia. *Archives of General Psychiatry*, **43**, 712–713.

GREEN, M. F., SATZ, P., SOPER, H. V., *et al* (1987) Relationship between physical anomalies and age of onset of schizophrenia. *American Journal of Psychiatry*, **144**, 666–667.

———, ———, GAIER, D. J., *et al* (1989) Minor physical anomalies in schizophrenia. *Schizophrenia Bulletin*, **15**, 91–99.

GROSSMAN, L. S., HARROW, M. & SANDS, J. R. (1986) Features associated with thought disorder in manic patients at 2 and 4 year follow-up. *American Journal of Psychiatry*, **143**, 306–311.

GUALTIERI, C. T., ADAMS, A., SHEN, C. D., *et al* (1982) Minor physical anomalies in alcoholic and schizophrenic adults and hyperactive and autistic children. *American Journal of Psychiatry*, **139**, 640–643.

GUY, J. D., MAJORSKI, L. V., WALLACE, C. J., *et al* (1983) The incidence of minor physical anomalies in adult male schizophrenics. *Schizophrenia Bulletin*, **9**, 571–582.

HAFNER, H., RIECHER, A., MAURER, K., *et al* (1989) How does gender influence age at first hospitalisation for schizophrenia? A transitional case register study. *Psychological Medicine*, **19**, 903–918.

HARDING, C. M., BROOKS, C., ASHIKAGA, T., *et al* (1987) The Vermont longitudinal study of persons with severe mental illness II: Long term outcome of subjects who retrospectively met DSMII criteria for schizophrenia. *American Journal of Psychiatry*, **144**, 727–735.

HARROW, M., GROSSMAN, L. S., SILVERSTEIN, M. L., *et al* (1982) Thought pathology in manic and schizophrenic patients: its occurrence at hospital admission and seven weeks later. *Archives of General Psychiatry*, **39**, 665–671.

HUBER, G., GROSS, G., SCHUTTLER, R., *et al* (1980) Longitudinal studies of schizophrenic patients. *Schizophrenia Bulletin*, **6**, 592–605.

JACOBY, R. J. & LEVY, R. (1980) Computed tomography in the elderly. 3. Affective disorder. *British Journal of Psychiatry*, **136**, 270–275.

JAKOB, H. & BECKMANN, H. (1986) Prenatal development disturbances in the limbic allocortex in schizophrenics. *Journal of Neural Transmission*, **65**, 303–326.

JESTE, D. V., LOHR, J. B. & GOODWIN, F. K. (1988) Neuroanatomical studies of major affective disorders: a review and suggestions for further research. *British Journal of Psychiatry*, **153**, 444–459.

JOHNSTONE, E. C., CROW, T. J., FRITH, C. D., *et al* (1976) Cerebral ventricular size and cognitive impairment in chronic schizophrenia. *Lancet*, *ii*, 924–926.

———, OWENS, D. G. C., CROW, T. J., *et al* (1989) Temporal lobe structure as determined by nuclear magnetic resonance in schizophrenia and bipolar affective disorder. *Journal of Neurology, Neurosurgery and Psychiatry*, **52**, 736–741.

JONES, P. & MURRAY, R. M. (1990) Aberrant neurodevelopment as the expression of the schizophrenia genotype. In *The New Genetics of Mental Illness* (eds P. McGuffin & R. M. Murray). London: Heinemann Medical Books.

KENDELL, R. & GOURLAY, J. (1970) The clinical distinction between the affective psychoses and schizophrenia. *British Journal of Psychiatry*, **117**, 261–266.

——— & BROCKINGTON, I. (1980) The identification of disease entities and the relationship between schizophrenic and affective psychoses. *British Journal of Psychiatry*, **137**, 324–330.

KENDLER, K. S. (1988) Familial aggregation of schizophrenia and schizophrenia spectrum disorders. *Archives of General Psychiatry*, **45**, 377–383.

—— & HAYS, P. (1983) Schizophrenia subdivided by the family history of affective disorder. *Archives of General Psychiatry*, **40**, 951–955.

—— & GRUENBERG, A. M. (1984) An independent analysis of the Danish adoption study of schizophrenia. VI. The relationship between psychiatric disorders as defined by DSMIII in the relatives of adoptees. *Archives of General Psychiatry*, **41**, 555–564.

——, ——, & TSUANG, M. T. (1985) Psychiatric illness in first degree relatives of schizophrenic and surgical control patients. *Archives of General Psychiatry*, **8**, 770–779.

KETY, S. S. (1980) The syndrome of schizophrenia: unresolved questions and opportunities for research. *British Journal of Psychiatry*, **136**, 421–426.

——, ROSENTHAL, D. & WENDER, D. H. (1978) Genetic relationships within the schizophrenic spectrum: evidence from adoption studies. In *Critical Issues in Psychiatric Diagnosis* (eds R. L. Spitzer & D. F. Klein). New York: River Press.

KOEHLER, K. (1979) First-rank symptoms of schizophrenia: questions concerning clinical boundaries. *British Journal of Psychiatry*, **134**, 236–248.

KOLAKOWSKA, T., WILLIAMS, A. O., ARDERN, M., *et al* (1985) Schizophrenia with good and poor outcome: 1. Early clinical features, response to neuroleptics and signs of organic dysfunction. *British Journal of Psychiatry*, **146**, 229–246.

KRAEPELIN, E. (1896) *Ein Lehrbuch Studirende end Acrzte*. Leipzig: Ambosius Berth.

—— (1913) *Dementia Praecox and Paraphrenia* (trans. 1919 from *Psychiatrie*, vol. III, part 2 (8th edn)). Edinburgh: E. & S. Livingstone.

KRETSCHMER, E. (1921) *Physique and Character: An Investigation of the Nature of Constitution and of the Theory of Temperament*. (Trans. E. Miller.) New York: Cooper Square Publishers.

LEE, A. S. & MURRAY, R. M. (1988) The long-term outcome of Maudsley depressives. *British Journal of Psychiatry*, **153**, 741–751.

LEWINE, R. R. J. (1981) Sex differences in schizophrenia: timing or subtypes? *Psychological Bulletin*, **90**, 432–444.

—— (1988) Gender and schizophrenia. In *Handbook of Schizophrenia. Vol. 3. Nosology, Epidemiology and Genetics* (eds M. Tsuang & J. Simpson). Amsterdam: Elsevier Press.

LEWIS, S. W. & MURRAY, R. M. (1987) Obstetric complications, neurodevelopmental deviance and risk of schizophrenia. *Journal of Psychiatric Research*, **21**, 413–422.

——, —— & OWEN, M. J. (1989) Obstetric complications in schizophrenia. Methodology and mechanisms. In *Schizophrenia: Scientific Progress* (eds S. C. Schultz & C. A. Tamminga). New York: Oxford University Press.

LINDENMEYER, J. P., KAY, S. R. & VAN PRAAG, H. M. (1989) Schizoaffective disorder: a distinct diagnostic entity. *Proceedings of the Annual Meeting of the American Psychiatric Association*, p. 305. Washington, DC: APA.

LORANGER, A. W. (1984) Sex differences in age at onset of schizophrenia. *Archives of General Psychiatry*, **41**, 157–161.

LUCHINS, D. J., LEWINE, R. J. & MELTZER, H. Y. (1983) Lateral ventricular size in the psychoses: relation to psychopathology and therapeutic and adverse response to medications. *Psychopharmacology Bulletin*, **19**, 518–522.

——, —— & —— (1984) Lateral ventricular size, psychopathology, and medication response in the psychoses. *Biological Psychiatry*, **19**, 29–44.

MARCUS, J., HANS, S. L., LEWOW, E., *et al* (1985) Neurological findings in high-risk children: childhood assessment and 5 year follow-up. *Schizophrenia Bulletin*, **11**, 85–100.

MAYER-GROSS, W. (1932) Die schizophrenia. In *Handbuch der Geistesk ranken Reiten Band IX* (ed. O. Bumke). Berlin: Springer.

McCABE, M. S., FOWLER, R. C., CADORET, R. J., *et al* (1971) Familial differences in schizophrenia with good and poor prognosis. *Psychological Medicine*, **1**, 326–332.

McGUFFIN, P., REVELEY, A. M. & HOLLAND, A. (1982) Identical triplets: non-identical psychosis? *British Journal of Psychiatry*, **140**, 1–6.

——, FARMER, A., GOTTESMAN, I. I., *et al* (1984) Twin concordance for operationally defined schizophrenia: confirmation of familiality and heritability. *Archives of General Psychiatry*, **41**, 541–545.

——, MURRAY, R. M. & REVELEY, A. M. (1987) Genetic influence on the psychoses. *British Medical Bulletin*, **43**, 531–556.

McNEIL, T. F. (1987) Perinatal influences in the development of schizophrenia. In *Biological Pespectives of Schizophrenia* (eds H. Helmehan & F. A. Henn). Bristol: John Wiley.

—— & KAIJ, L. (1978) Obstetric factors in the development of schizophrenia. In *The Nature of Schizophrenia* (eds L. C. Wynne, R. L. Cromwell & S. Matthysse). New York: John Wiley.

MELLOR, C. S. (1970) First rank symptoms of schizophrenia. *British Journal of Psychiatry*, **117**, 15–23.

MURRAY, R. M., REVELEY, A. M. & CLIFFORD, C. A. (1984) The contribution of genetics to psychiatric nosology. Paper presented at the Plenary Session of the Congress of the World Psychiatric Association, Vienna, Austria.

MURRAY, R. M., LEWIS, S. W., REVELEY, A. M. (1985) Towards an aetiological classification of schizophrenia. *Lancet*, *i*, 1023–1026.

——, REVELEY, A. M. & McGUFFIN, P. (1986) Genetic vulnerability to schizophrenia. In *Schizophrenia* (ed. A. Roy). *Psychiatric Clinics of North America*, **9**, 3–16.

——, LEWIS, S. W., OWEN, M. J., *et al* (1988) The neurodevelopmental origins of dementia praecox. In *Schizophrenia The Major Issues* (eds P. McGuffin & P. Bebbington). London: Heinemann.

NYBACK, H., WEISEL, F. A., BERGGREN, B. M., *et al* (1982) Computed tomography of the brain in patients with acute psychosis and healthy volunteers. *Acta Psychiatrica Scandinavica*, **65**, 403–414.

ØDEGÅRD, Ø. (1972) The multifactorial inheritance of predisposition to schizophrenia. In *Genetic Factors in Schizophrenia* (ed. A. R. Kaplan). Springfield: C. C. Thomas.

OWEN, M. J., LEWIS, S. W. & MURRAY, R. M. (1988) Obstetric complications and schizophrenia: a computed tomographic study. *Psychological Medicine*, **18**, 331–339.

PAYKEL, E. & WEISSMAN, M. M. (1973) Social adjustment and depression. A longitudinal study. *Archives of General Psychiatry*, **28**, 659–663.

PEARLSON, G. D., GARBACZ, D. J., BREAKEY, W. R., *et al* (1984*a*) Lateral ventricular enlargement associated with persistent unemployment and negative symptoms in both schizophrenia and bipolar disorder. *Psychiatry Research*, **12**, 1–9.

——, ——, TOMPKINS, R. H., *et al* (1984*b*) Clinical correlates of lateral ventricular enlargement in bipolar affective disorder. *American Journal of Psychiatry*, **141**, 253–256.

——, KIM, W. S. & KUBOS, K. L. (1989) Ventricular brain ratio, computed tomographic density and brain area in 50 schizophrenics. *Archives of General Psychiatry*, **46**, 690–697.

POPE, H. G. & LIPINSKI, J. F. (1978) Diagnosis in schizophrenia and manic depressive illness: a reassessment of the specificity of "schizophrenic" symptoms in the light of current research. *Archives of General Psychiatry*, **35**, 811–828.

ROBERTS, G. W., COLTER, N., LOFTHOUSE, R., *et al* (1987) Is there gliosis in schizophrenia? Investigation of the temporal lobe. *Biological Psychiatry*, **22**, 1459–1468.

ROY-BYRNE, P. P., POST, R. M., KELLNER, C. H., *et al* (1988) Ventricular brain ratio and life course of illness in patients with affective disorder. *Psychiatry Research*, **23**, 277–284.

SACCHETTI, E., VITA, A., CONTE, G., *et al* (1987) Brain morphology in major affective disorders: clinical and biological correlates. In *Proceedings of the International Meeting on Plasticity and Morphology of the Central Nervous System*. Milan, pp. 49–51. Lancaster: MTP Press.

SCHARFETTER, C. & NUSPERLI, M. (1980) The group of schizophrenias, schizoaffective psychoses and affective disorders. *Schizophrenia Bulletin*, **65**, 586–591.

SHETTAR, S. M., ARAVAPALLI, R., HASKETT, R. F., *et al* (1990) Limbic measures by MRI in depressives and controls. *Proceedings of the 143rd Annual Meeting of the American Psychiatric Association. May 12–17*. Washington, DC: American Psychiatric Press.

SHIMA, S., SHIKANO, T., KITAMURA, R., *et al* (1984) Depression and ventricular enlargement. *Acta Psychiatrica Scandinavica*, **70**, 275–277.

SMITH, D. W. (1976) *Recognisable Patterns of Human Malformation: Genetic, Embryological and Clinical Aspects*. Philadelphia: W. B. Saunders.

SPITZER, R. L., ENDICOTT, J. R. & ROBINS, E. (1978) *Research Diagnostic Criteria (RDC) for a Selected Group of Functional Disorders* (3rd edn). New York: New York State Psychiatric Institute.

ST CLAIR, D., BLACKWOOD, D., MUIR, W., *et al* (1989) No linkage of chromosome 5 q11-13 markers to schizophrenia in Scottish families. *Nature*, **339**, 305–309.

STANDISH-BARRY, H. M. A. S., BOURAS, N., BRIDGES, P. K., *et al* (1982) Pneumo-encephalographic and computerised axial tomography scan changes in affective disorders. *British Journal of Psychiatry*, **141**, 614–617.

SUDDATH, R. L., CASANOVA, M. D., GOLDBERG, T. E., *et al* (1989) Temporal lobe pathology in schizophrenia: a quantitative magnetic resonance imaging study. *American Journal of Psychiatry*, **146**, 464–472.

TARGUM, S. D., ROSEN, L. M., DELISI, L. E., *et al* (1983) Cerebral ventricular size in major depressive disorder: association with delusional symptoms. *Biological Psychiatry*, **18**, 329–336.

WADDINGTON, J. L. & YOUSSEF, H. (1988) The expression of schizophrenia, affective disorder and vulnerability to tardive dyskinesia in an extensive pedigree. *British Journal of Psychiatry*, **153**, 376–381.

——, O'CALLAGHAN, E. & LARKIN, E. (1990) Physical anomalies and neurodevelopmental abnormality in schizophrenia: new clinical correlates. *Schizophrenia Research*, **3**, 90.

WEINBERGER, D. R., CANNON-SPOOR, E., POTKIN, S. G., *et al* (1980) Poor premorbid adjustment and CT scan abnormalities in chronic schizophrenia. *American Journal of Psychiatry*, **137**, 1410–1413.

——, DELISI, L. E., PERMAN, G. P., *et al* (1982) Computed tomography in schizophreniform disorder and other psychiatric disorders. *Archives of General Psychiatry*, **39**, 778–783.

WILCOX, J. A. & NASRALLAH, H. A. (1987) Perinatal distress and prognosis of psychotic illness. *Neuropsychobiology*, **17**, 173–175.

WILLIAMS, A. O., REVELEY, M. A., KOLAKOWSKA, T., *et al* (1985) Schizophrenia with good and poor outcome: II Cerebral ventricular size and its clinical significance. *British Journal of Psychiatry*, **146**, 239–246.

WING, J. & NIXON, J. (1975) Discriminating symptoms in schizophrenia. *Archives of General Psychiatry*, **32**, 853–859.

WOODS, B. T., KINNEY, D. K. & YURGELUN-TODD, D. (1986) Neurologic abnormalities in schizophrenic patients and their families. I. Comparison of schizophrenic, bipolar and substance abuse patients and normal controls. *Archives of General Psychiatry*, **43**, 657–663.

——, YURGELUN-TODD, D. & KINNEY, D. K. (1987) Relationship of neurological abnormalities in schizophrenics to family psychopathology. *Biological Psychiatry*, **21**, 325–331.

5 Affective symptoms in schizophrenia, basic, prodromal and residual: implications for a functional approach to diagnosis

STEVEN R. HIRSCH

A double-blind withdrawal study of the efficacy of depot medication in schizophrenia has found that a substantial proportion of chronic schizophrenics required treatment with antidepressants during the trial (Hirsch *et al*, 1973). The number was higher in the group who had placebo substituted for fluphenazine depot injections during the nine months of the study. The World Health Organization's (1973) report on the International Pilot Study of Schizophrenia revealed almost as high a prevalence rate of depressive symptoms in recently admitted schizophrenics as in patients diagnosed with psychotic or neurotic depression – approximately 80% of the schizophrenics had ''simple depression'' or ''other symptoms of depression'' compared with 76% of those with mania or 97% of patients with depression.

Subsequently Knights and I studied a year's cohort of acute admissions to an outer London borough of 90 000 population (Knights & Hirsch, 1981). Figure 5.1 shows the proportion of all patients who could be interviewed

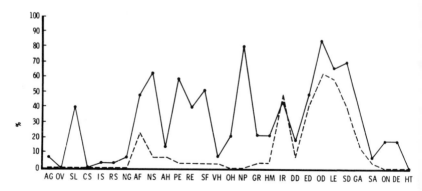

Fig. 5.1. *Percentage of 27 acute admissions to a psychiatric unit who had scored + or + + for syndromes on the Present State Examination at admission (——) and after three months (----). Affective and neurotic symptoms appear towards the right, schizophrenic and psychotic symptoms towards the left (OD, other symptoms of depression; SD, simple depression; NS, nuclear schizophrenia; NP, non-specific psychosis) (from Knights & Hirsch, 1981)*

and who had depressive syndromes on the Present State Examination (PSE; Wing *et al*, 1974) at the time of admission and three months later. Affective and neurotic symptoms were present in more than 70% of patients. Interestingly, three months later depressive symptoms were shown to persist but nearly all patients had lost their schizophrenic and other psychotic symptoms. In the same study we showed that the 62 admissions for depression and neurosis during the same year had a slightly higher incidence of depressive and neurotic symptoms when admitted to hospital – 90–100% – but the difference between depressives and schizophrenics three months after admission was negligible.

Other workers have reported similar high rates of depression and affective symptoms in schizophrenia, and studies of acute admissions have shown the point prevalence to be highest during the acute phase and to diminish as the patients recover. For example, Moller & Von Zerssen (1981) studied 280 patients recently admitted with schizophrenia and found 48% had depressive symptoms on admission but only 14% when patients were discharged. Only 16% developed depressive symptoms who did not have depression at the time of admission. The finding that depressive symptoms have their highest prevalence at the acute phase of the illness and tend to diminish in prevalence but recur at intervals throughout the illness is now well established (Knights *et al*, 1979; Johnson, 1981; Jolley *et al*, 1989).

The earlier findings have been confirmed in a five-year follow-up report from the Rhine Necker cohort study, a prospective study reported by Biehl *et al* (1988). Using the PSE, they assessed 70 patients who had had the onset of illness within the previous year and followed them with six-monthly assessments for two years and follow-up assessments at years 3 and 5. Using the four CATEGO subscales for non-specific neurotic symptoms, specific neurotic symptoms, behavioural speech and other psychotic syndromes, and delusional and hallucinatory syndromes, the group of non-specific neurotic symptoms had the highest score at every assessment; delusional and hallucinatory symptoms had the lowest score except at first assessment, during the acute phase. Examining the relative proportion of CATEGO symptom classes present at each of the seven assessments, affective and neurotic symptoms constituted more than half the CATEGO syndromes identified at each of the assessments from six months to five years. Factor analysis of the PSE syndromes identified a delusional factor, an anxiety factor, and a residual affective factor for which the strongest loadings were tiredness or exhaustion, subjective inefficient thinking, neglect due to brooding, loss of interest, depressed mood, hopelessness, morning depression, self-depreciation, lack of confidence, subjective anergy and retardation, loss of libido and lost emotions.

The conclusion one can draw from these studies is that affective symptoms make up a substantial part of the schizophrenic symptom pattern, being present in approximately half of all schizophrenics during an acute admission and at some time during the six months following admission (Knights *et al*, 1979). Although they very slowly become less prevalent over time, Johnson's two-year follow-up found that 70% of chronic schizophrenics show significant depressive symptoms at some time during two years following an acute episode, and this is consistent with the findings of Biehl *et al* (1988). At the same time one should note that in chronic 'back-ward' schizophrenics, depressive symptoms can be differentiated from the residual symptoms of chronic schizophrenia and depressive symptoms are in fact relatively rare, with a prevalence of about 10% (Hirsch *et al*, 1989).

Affective symptoms as prodromes to acute schizophrenic relapse

Our understanding of the relationship between affective symptoms and schizophrenia was extended in a new direction when Herz & Melville (1980) studied the symptoms which precede, or are prodromal to, a schizophrenic relapse. Two large cohorts of patients and their relatives were asked what symptoms were present before the reappearance of symptoms specific to schizophrenia. The long list of neurotic and depressive symptoms which emerged was fairly consistent across both cohorts, which together comprised 180 patients. A prospective study by Gross (1989) in which prodromal symptoms were the trigger for a brief treatment intervention intended to suppress an impending relapse found a similar profile of prodromal symptoms. In Herz's study more than 70% of patients reported nervousness and tenseness as a prodrome to schizophrenic symptoms and more than 60% reported impaired concentration, sleep disturbance, restlessness, depression, reduced enjoyment, and preoccupation with one or two things. Half experienced loss of interest and ideas of reference. There are a host of other neurotic or depressive symptoms which have been reported in both studies in a descending order of frequency.

Our study (Jolley *et al*, 1989) is one of four which have investigated the hypothesis that affective symptoms are a part of schizophrenia, which emerge early during the reactivation which precedes relapse, and can be used to trigger a treatment intervention with neuroleptics to prevent relapse. Our hypothesis was that if affective symptoms are prodromal to a symptom of relapse and an inherent part of the schizophrenic process, they would be expected to precede a relapse more frequently in patients who have been switched from depot medication to a placebo injection, than in patients who continue on depot phenothiazines. In the first year of follow-up, admittedly during which depot neuroleptics continued to be present in decreasing concentrations in the body, 76% of the placebo patients compared with 27% of the controls experienced prodromal symptoms. All the patients were treated immediately with 5–10 mg of haloperidol daily and almost all showed a reduction in the symptoms back to baseline within two weeks. This suggests but does not prove that affective symptoms of schizophrenia are held in check by neuroleptics and emerge when neuroleptics are withdrawn. Whether the remission that was observed on oral haloperidol supplements would have occurred spontaneously had patients not received haloperidol needs to be tested in a prospective study. Such studies are in fact in progress under the auspices of the National Institutes of Health in the USA.

It should be noted that the concept that non-specific affective symptoms are an inherent part of the disease process and are even more basic to the schizophrenia process than the florid symptoms of hallucinations and delusions can be traced back to Bleuler, but has had strong representation in more recent times by Huber (1983) and Gross (1989).

Cross-over between treatment modalities for schizophrenia and depression

Although we often like to think otherwise, the concept that depression responds to antidepressants and schizophrenia responds to neuroleptics is not as clear cut as we might like to believe. Antipsychotic neuroleptics such as thioridazine, fluphenazine and more recently flupenthixol have been shown to be effective in the treatment of at least mild and moderate depression. For example, Young *et al* (1976) carried out a double-blind comparison of flupenthixol and amitriptyline in mild and moderate out-patient cases of depression and found them to be equally effective. Paykel & Coppen (1968) have reviewed the problem and found a number of studies which support this finding using different neuroleptics in the treatment of schizophrenia.

One explanation is that neuroleptics in low doses increase the outflow of pre-synaptic dopamine by selectively blocking pre-synaptic dopamine autoreceptors. If this were the case, the efficacy of neuroleptics in the treatment of depression would not really support the concept that the two conditions overlap, because we would be talking about different dosage levels and different mechanisms of action to explain the treatment effect.

There is also evidence that shows that lithium is effective in the treatment of schizophrenia-like psychoses, but the effect is mainly an anti-excitation effect in patients who are overactive or who have a mixed affective disorder (Hirsch, 1986). The efficacy of antidepressants in the treatment of schizophrenia is a more complicated issue because one has to separate out the effects of antidepressants on such schizophrenic symptoms as slowness and retardation, which may be confused with depressive symptoms, from true antidepressant effects in patients who already have a depressive syndrome as well as a schizophrenic illness. Most studies fail to show a significant antidepressive effect, but more recently Sirus *et al* (1987) published a well controlled study of schizophrenic patients who had a depressive syndrome which would by itself qualify as major depression by DSM–III criteria (American Psychiatric Association, 1980). They showed a significant beneficial effect of amitriptyline over placebo when added to ongoing neuroleptic treatment in schizophrenic patients who had a full-blown depressive syndrome. Finally it should be mentioned that electroconvulsive therapy (ECT), although often thought only to be effective in catatonic schizophrenia, is in fact very effective in the treatment of acute florid schizophrenia. The evidence of both well designed placebo-controlled studies and large less well controlled studies is reviewed elsewhere (Hirsch, 1986).

Should we be forced into the Procrustean bed of current diagnostic practice?

Where does this discussion lead us? As psychiatrists raised in the Kraepelinian tradition, we feel there are important and useful distinctions to be made between schizophrenia and the affective psychoses which are relevant to treatment and prognosis. It is clear that affective symptoms are an inherent part of the schizophrenic syndrome. Johnson (1981) followed up 30 chronic schizophrenics over two years in the community, assessing them monthly as to whether they had sufficient symptoms to be independently diagnosed as depressed or not. He found that 60% of such patients experienced at least one episode of depressive illness, as judged by a rating scale (Hamilton or Beck), at some time during this period. Depression alone was responsible for 70% of the patients' morbidity measured in weeks over the two years, while only 30% could be ascribed to schizophrenic symptoms alone or schizophrenic symptoms plus depression (Liddle & Barnes, 1990). On the other hand, because of the hierarchical way we make diagnoses, schizophrenic symptoms are not very prevalent in depressive syndromes because we make the diagnosis of schizophrenia when they occur. Nevertheless, the overlap between the two syndromes is undeniable.

The advances of modern technology in neuropsychophysiology, including brain mapping using electroencephalography, and metabolic imaging techniques such as single-photon emission computerised tomography (SPECT) and positron emission tomography (PET) are beginning to give us results which I think may force a different approach. They suggest that focusing on symptoms and syndromes as the basic entity of observation may be a more useful strategy than trying to elucidate the underlying mechanisms in the pathophysiology of these disorders. For example, Liddle & Barnes (1990) have factor analysed the symptoms of a cohort of chronic schizophrenic patients with unremitting refractory symptoms. This is a group of special interest because the persisting nature of the symptoms should make the identification of underlying pathophysiological abnormalities easier to detect. The factor analysis showed a consistent pattern, with three basic factors emerging: (a) a psychomotor poverty syndrome, with poverty of speech, poverty of movement, poverty of expression, and lack of responsiveness; (b) a disorganisation syndrome, with inappropriate affect, tangentiality of speech, derailment of speech, pressure of speech, distractability; and (c) a reality distortion syndrome, with chronic delusions. Current research in our department is based on the hypothesis that these syndromes represent separate pathophysiological disturbances relevant respectively to the dorsolateral pre-frontal cortex, the orbital miatal frontal cortex, and the hypothalamus or hippocampus. This approach is based on the findings of previous authors, such as Kleist, that lesions in the dorsolateral pre-frontal cortex cause a syndrome not dissimilar from Liddle's psychomotor poverty syndrome, while orbital miatal lesions cause a syndrome similar to the disorganisation syndrome.

Elsewhere I have reviewed supporting evidence from Weinberger and from Kashimoto which would associate a psychomotor poverty syndrome with frontal lobe abnormalities (Hirsch, 1988). A functional approach such as this one helps to explain the disparity of results from different centres using computerised tomography and PET techniques. Centres such as ours, which have reported normal frontal lobe function in schizophrenia, focus their studies on patients with acute Schneiderian positive schizophrenia in the absence of chronic negative symptoms. Most centres however have studied chronic patients with predominantly negative symptoms, who show a high prevalence of psychomotor poverty syndrome, thereby explaining hypometabolism in the frontal lobes (Gruzelier *et al*, 1988).

O'Connel *et al* (personal communication) from the USA using SPECT found decreased cerebral blood flow was inversely related to high scores on the Hamilton Rating Scale for Depression, regardless of diagnosis. Frontal lobe blood flow was reduced in patients who were withdrawn, whether they were schizophrenic or had retarded depression. Hypothalamic blood flow was increased in patients with hallucinations and delusions regardless of diagnosis, which included schizophrenia, depression and mania. These findings are consistent with the Liddle hypothesis outlined above.

Gruzelier & Manchanda (1982) studied the lateralisation of the galvanic skin-orienting response. They analysed symptom ratings on the PSE and the Brief Psychiatric Rating Scale in acute newly admitted schizophrenics, all of whom had Schneider's first-rank symptoms – hence they were very different from the refractory group described by Liddle and Barnes. Galvanic skin response to a moderate-intensity 100 Hz 70 dB tone distinguished two groups of patients within this acute, Schneiderian-positive schizophrenic group, in one of which the orienting response was deficient on the right side (the 'active syndrome'), in the other of which the orienting response was deficient on the left side (the 'withdrawn syndrome'). Thus a group of symptoms drawn from standardised rating scales correlated with the localised functional change involving lateralisation of the orientating response (Gaebel *et al*, 1986). Gaebel *et al* also examined eye tracking of these two groups of patients with a visual search test in which they had to identify a 'Z' which was laid out in a maze of 285 randomised letters of the alphabet. Patients with a decreased left-hemisphere function took a *Gestalt* or 'parallel processing' approach, which enabled them to move rapidly to define the correct letter without scanning cross-wise in reading fashion. Normal subjects tended to scan across left to right, and took significantly longer.

When one examines the neurophysiological functioning of the 'active' and 'withdrawn' groups one finds a worse performance on the Warrington Recognition of Faces test in the active group compared with normal controls, while the withdrawn group show a worse performance in the Word Recognition Test. The active group were normal on the Word Recognition Test and the withdrawn group were normal in the Faces Test (Gruzelier, 1990). Elizabeth Warrington at the National Hospital, Queen Square, had developed the Faces Recognition and Word Recognition tests using brain-damaged patients and found that patients with right temporoparietal lesions performed poorly on the faces test while patients with left temporoparietal lesions performed poorly on the word recognition test (Warrington, 1984).

Conclusion

In reporting these results I have knowingly skirted around the central question, whether schizophrenia and depression are one illness or two. I have done this in order to illustrate the point that progress may depend more on relating our investigations to underlying disturbances of function and subsets of clinical phenomena, than relating them to diagnostic groups. This does not deny the usefulness, from a clinical point of view, of a diagnostic approach which serves clinicians well, but does so at the risk of obscuring the considerable overlap between the diagnostic entities of neurotic and psychotic depressive and schizophrenic syndromes. It does so at the risk of obscuring important relationships between function and structure, and clinical phenomena. This may best be identified by looking at the symptoms and syndromes that different diagnostic groups have in common. I suggest that this will prove to be a more profitable approach for progress in understanding the neurobiological basis of psychiatry.

References

AMERICAN PSYCHIATRIC ASSOCIATION (1980) *Diagnostic and Statistical Manual of Mental Disorders* (3rd edn) (DSM–III). Washington, DC: APA.
BIEHL, H., MAURER, K., JUNG, E., *et al* (1988) Reported symptoms in schizophrenic patients

within 5 years of onset of illness. In *Treatment of Refractory Schizophrenia* (eds S. J. Dencker & F. Kulhanek), pp. 108–118. Braunschweig: Vieweg.

GAEBEL, W., ULRICH, G. & FRICK, K. (1986) Eye-movement research with schizophrenic patients and normal controls using corneal reflection-pupil centre measurement. *European Archives of Psychiatry and Neurological Sciences*, **236**, 243–254.

GROSS, G. (1989) The "basic" symptoms of schizophrenia. *British Journal of Psychiatry*, **155** (suppl. 7), 21–25.

GRUZELIER, J. H. (1990) Brain localisation and neuropsychology in schizophrenia: syndrome and neurodevelopmental implications. In *Search for the Causes of Schizophrenia II* (eds H.Hafner & W. F. Gattaz). Berlin: Springer Verlag.

—— & MANCHANDA, R. (1982) The syndrome of schizophrenia: relations between electrodermal response, lateral asymmetries and clinical ratings. *British Journal of Psychiatry*, **141**, 485–488.

——, SEYMOUR, K., WILSON, L., *et al* (1988) Impairments on neurological tests of temporohippocampal and fronto-hippocampal functions and word fluency in remitting schizophrenia and affective disorders. *Archives of General Psychiatry*, **45**, 623–629.

HERZ, M. & MELVILLE, C. (1980) Relapse in schizophrenia. *American Journal of Psychiatry*, **137**, 801–805.

HIRSCH, S. R. (1982) Depression "revealed" in schizophrenia. *British Journal of Psychiatry*, **140**, 421–424.

—— (1986) The treatment of schizophrenia. In *The Psychopharmacology and Treatment of Schizophrenia* (eds P. Bradley & S. R. Hirsch). Oxford: Oxford University Press.

—— (1988) Essential aspects of the research problem in schizophrenia. *Journal of the Royal Society of Medicine*, **81**, 691–697.

——, GAIND, R., ROHDE, P. D., *et al* (1973) Outpatient maintenance of chronic schizophrenic patients with long-acting fluphenazine: double blind placebo trial. *British Medical Journal*, i, 633–637.

——, JOLLEY, A. G., BARNES, T. R. E., *et al* (1989) Dysphoric and depressive symptoms in chronic schizophrenia. *Schizophrenia Research*, **2**, 259–264.

HUBER, G. (1983) Das Konzept substratnaber Baissymptome und seine Bedutung für Therapie bei und Therapie schizophrenen Erkrankunger. *Nervenartz*, **54**, 23–32.

JOHNSON, D. A. W. (1981) Studies of depressive symptoms in schizophrenia. *British Journal of Psychiatry*, **139**, 89–101.

JOLLEY, A. G., HIRSCH, S. R., McRINK, A., *et al* (1989) Trial of brief intermittent prophylaxis for selected schizophrenic outpatients: clinical outcome at one year. *British Medical Journal*, **298**, 985–990.

KNIGHTS, A., OKASHA, M. S., SALEH, M. A., *et al* (1979) Depressive and extrapyramidal symptoms and clinical effects: a trial of fluphenazine versus flupenthixol in maintenance of schizophrenic outpatients. *British Journal of Psychiatry*, **135**, 515–523.

—— & HIRSCH, S. R. (1981) "Revealed" depression drug treatment. *Archives of General Psychiatry*, **38**, 806–811.

LIDDLE, P. F. & BARNES, T. R. E. (1990) Symptoms of chronic schizophrenia. *British Journal of Psychiatry*, **157**, 558–561.

MOLLER, H. J. & VON ZERSSEN, D. (1981) Depressive Symptomatik im Stationaren Behandlungsverlauf von 280 schizophrenen Patienten. *Pharmacopsychiatria*, **14**, 172–179.

PAYKEL, E. & COPPEN, A. (1968) *Psychopharmacology of Affective Disorders*, pp. 208–209. Oxford: Oxford University Press.

SIRUS, S. G., MORGAN, V., FAGERSTROM, R., *et al* (1987) Adjunctive imipramine in the treatment of post-psychotic depression: a controlled trial. *Archives of General Psychiatry*, **44**, 533–539.

WARRINGTON, E. K. (1984) *Recognition Memory Test*. Windsor: NFER-Nelson.

WING, J. K., COOPER, J. E. & SARTORIUS, N. (1974) *The Description and Classification of Psychiatric Syndromes*. London: Cambridge University Press.

WORLD HEALTH ORGANIZATION (1973) *Report of the International Pilot Study of Schizophrenia*, B3, B22, C7. Geneva: WHO.

YOUNG, J. P. R., HUGHES, W. C. & LADER, M. H. (1976) A controlled comparison of flupenthixol and amitriptyline in depressed outpatients. *British Medical Journal*, i, 1116–1118.

6 An American perspective on the conceptual approaches to psychopathology

GERALD L. KLERMAN

The debate over the relative values of dimensional versus categorical approaches to psychopathology has continued over a number of decades (Lorr, 1986). One might have expected that this debate was a purely technical statistical issue and would have been resolved by appropriate expert involvement by biostatisticians. Indeed, there have been many studies involving the use of multivariate statistics in attempting to resolve this debate. However, it appears that in addition to technical statistical issues a number of extra-statistical issues are involved in this debate, issues that have to do with the nature of mental illness, the status of psychiatry as a medical specialty, and the role of mental illness and mental health in the larger society (Rothblum *et al*, 1986; Mirowsky & Ross, 1989; Klerman, 1990*a*).

In general, proponents of categorical approaches tend to be psychiatrists, often with strong biological orientation, who emphasise that psychiatry is a specialty of medicine. They point out that, in psychiatry as in most of medicine, most important clinical decisions are binary – To admit to hospital or not? To start a treatment? To stop a treatment? To discharge into the community? Clinicians prefer diagnostic categories that will justify difficult clinical and social decisions and consequently they prefer typologies and groupings rather than dimensions.

In contrast, the proponents of dimensional approaches tend to be psychologists and biostatisticians, but also include a large number of psychiatrists concerned with psychological and behavioural causes and treatments of mental illness. They are often critical, if not suspicious, of biological treatments such as drugs or electroconvulsive therapy (Klerman, 1991). They regard dimensional approaches as more consistent with moral respect for the patient and minimising the social control exercised by psychiatrists who, it is claimed, justify their power and authority by involving the medical model (Szasz, 1974).

This chapter reviews the categorical versus dimensional controversy from the historical and conceptual perspective of US experience since World War II (Klerman, 1986, 1990*a*).

Historical development

There have been significant shifts in the dominant US approaches to psychiatry since World War II. Currently, the leadership in American academic and scientific psychiatric circles gives strong endorsement to the 'medical model', to biological psychiatry, and to the potential of neuroscience to contribute to better understanding and treatment of psychiatric disorders. These views have not always been as dominant as they are now and it is valuable to reconstruct the changes in paradigm since World War II, particularly as they relate to thinking about the concepts of mental illness and of diagnosis (Klerman, 1990*b*).

The paradigm shift

Psychiatric thinking, research, and clinical practice concerning issues of psychopathology, diagnosis and classification, underwent a major paradigm shift in the 1970s, culminating in the publication of DSM–III (American Psychiatric Association, 1980). The concept of 'paradigm shift' derives from the writings of Thomas Kuhn (1970), the historian and philosopher of science, who describes the history of a scientific field as punctuated by revolutions – periods in which there are major changes in the discipline's ideas, methods and social structure. During these revolutions, the dominant mode of thinking within the field changes. Kuhn refers to these modes of thinking as 'paradigms'. A paradigm has two components: cognitive (ideas, beliefs, and concepts) and communal (the group of scientists sharing a common point of view). This 'paradigm shift' in US psychiatry represented the success of what I have labelled the 'neo-Kraepelinian revival' (Klerman, 1978, 1990*a*). The essential tenet of the neo-Kraepelinian paradigm is that psychiatry (Klerman, 1977; Spitzer & Endicott, 1978) is the specialty of medicine concerned with mental disorders, with the scientific understanding of these disorders, and with the diagnosis and treatment of individuals suffering from them. The theory and measurement of these disorders utilises a categorical approach. The criteria for assigning individuals to diagnostic categories is based on algorithms, which should be based, wherever possible, on operationally defined, observable manifestations of psychopathology, with minimal inferences as to presumed causation. The neo-Kraepelinian approach proposes a limited scope of psychiatry, in reaction to the social psychiatry school which had advocated an expansion of psychiatry's scope during the community mental health era.

The impact of World War II on psychiatric thinking

The mental health experiences of the 'selective service system' and the armed forces during World War II were to have an important impact on psychiatry after the war. The selective service system rejected large numbers of young men for psychiatric reasons during World War II: neuropsychiatric conditions accounted for the largest proportion of rejections. It is of note that these psychiatric rejections included many individuals who were mild or moderately mentally retarded and also many who were mentally ill or emotionally troubled, or both. The scientific accuracy and validity of the diagnostic procedures were questioned; nevertheless, the publicity given to the high rates of mental retardation, psychoneurosis, personality disorders and psychosomatic illnesses focused public attention on mental health problems and supported the post-war efforts to obtain more information on rates of psychiatric disability.

Neuropsychiatric medical specialists were widely dispersed in the military medical services and contributed clinical descriptions of mental disorders related to combat and military service – such as combat fatigue, transient functional psychoses, dissociative states, and stress reactions. Statistical studies were also undertaken (Glass, 1958). Whereas the rates of psychoses in the military remained relatively stable, the rates of psychoneuroses and personality reactions fluctuated and were related to combat and other stresses, such as the extreme deprivation in prisoner of war (POW) camps and concentration camps.

In the army, a group of talented social scientists were organised (Stouffer *et al*, 1949). Using the best available sampling methods, survey techniques and statistical analyses, this group conducted a range of studies and developed neuropsychiatric screening questionnaires to relate neurotic symptoms to combat stress and morale problems. These scales were similar to the impairment scales used in community surveys after the war.

The observation that rates of psychiatric reactions varied in relation to combat stress was of practical utility and theoretical importance. These reactions to stress occurred in psychiatrically screened young men for whom pre-existing disability factors would seem to have been absent. From today's vantage point, these methods for screening and assessment were far from ideal. Nevertheless, their implications for studies after the war were highly important.

The leaders of US psychiatry after World War II were impressed by the selective service and military experience and concluded that precipitating stress, rather than predisposition or vulnerability, was the major factor in the causation of psychiatric illness. The role of stress as an immediate precipitant of mental illness was supported powerfully by these observations, and 'stress' was to be a major unifying concept in the post-war psychiatric studies in civilian settings. Poverty, urban anomie, rapid social change, and social class were to become the civilian stressors equivalent to combat for military personnel and threat of death for prisoners of war and those in Nazi concentration camps.

Later developments

After World War II, the experience gained by the military and the growing public awareness of the high prevalence of mental illness prompted epidemiological studies in the general population. There was financial and policy support for community surveys after the National Institute of Mental Health (NIMH) was created by Congress in 1946.

The decades after World War II became the 'golden era' of social epidemiology (Weissman & Klerman, 1978, 1984). The social epidemiological research undertaken in this 'golden era' was guided by the paradigm of social psychiatry. Investigators focused on large social institutions and historical forces such as urbanisation and industrialisation to understand the variations in prevalence of distress and disability. Studies representative of this period were: the Midtown Manhattan survey, which assessed the impact of urban life on mental health by interviewing more than 1000 adult residents selected by probability sampling in midtown Manhattan (Srole *et al*, 1962); the nationwide survey of mental health by Gurin *et al* (1960) of the University of Michigan Survey Research Center, in which more than 2000 adult Americans, also selected by probability sampling, were interviewed; and the cross-cultural studies of Leighton and associates that were undertaken in the 1950s in Nigeria, northern Canada, and the south-western United States after Leighton's research on Japanese–American internees in California during World War II. The well known Canadian community study by Leighton *et al* (1963) assessed the impact of social and economic change on the mental health of a previously stable rural community in Stirling, Nova Scotia. These studies all reported high rates of lifetime mental impairment. For example, the Midtown Manhattan study found that only 19% of the subjects were free of significant symptoms and that 23% were substantially impaired. Their rates were surprising and contributed to controversy over the validity of the study.

Hollingshead & Redlich (1958) investigated prevalence patterns of treated mental disorders in New Haven, Connecticut, establishing social class as an important determinant of prevalence of treated mental illness, particularly of schizophrenia. Their results were replicated by Myers & Bean (1968) who followed up the New Haven sample 10 years later. Weissman *et al* (1987) give a detailed account by the investigators of these studies, their purposes, methods and results.

These epidemiological studies had a number of important similarities. They gave detailed attention to the modes of selection and completeness of their samples. They decided against using existing psychiatric nosology out of concern for diagnostic unreliability; they substituted measures of overall mental impairment for traditional diagnostic categories. The use of general impairment scales rather than diagnostic judgements made it easier and more economical to execute surveys (Langner, 1962). Trained psychiatrists were no longer required to make diagnostic judgements: unreliability of diagnosis and nosological disputes could be avoided.

Many of the social scientists and psychiatrists conducting these studies explicitly rejected the traditional medical model of multiple separate psychiatric disorders due to diverse but specific causes. In this respect, there was considerable difference between the American approach after World War II and the approach adopted in Continental Europe and in Scandinavia. The Continental European and Scandinavian studies maintained the tradition of Kraepelin. Their use of traditional psychiatric diagnostic categories was based on the assumption that each illness had a different underlying aetiology, symptom pattern, course and response to treatment, and that biological (genetic, biochemical) factors, rather than social and environmental stress, most likely would explain the causes of different illnesses, at least for the major psychoses.

Mental health and mental illness, it was postulated, fell along a gradient. The most succinct expression of this viewpoint was offered by the National Advisory Mental Health Council (1955):

"The concept of etiology as embraced by modern psychiatry differs from the simple cause and effect system of traditional medicine. It subscribes to a 'field theory' hypothesis in which the interactions and transactions of multiple factors eventuate in degrees of health and sickness."

Among the multiple factors, genetics, birth defects, nutrition, infection, or biological variations were of lesser interest as possible causal agents than social class or stress.

A unitary concept of mental health as proposed by the National Advisory Mental Health Council was consistent with an emphasis on investigating social causes of mental illness. This unitary approach emphasised the importance of life experience in the understanding of the psychopathology of individuals and the role of economics, social class, and social stress in the aetiology of mental disorders. Diagnostic groups were considered merely quantitatively different manifestations of the same causes of mental functioning; common aetiological factors, social stressors, were considered to underlie psychiatric disorders.

Although the epidemiological surveys of the 1950s and the '60s generated a considerable body of information on mental health and impairment in the United States, those studies had serious limitations. Most important, they did not provide rates of specific psychiatric disorders. The impairment rates that were reported were independent of diagnosis and obscured diagnostic variations. Impairment rates could not be translated into equivalent clinical diagnostic categories. As a consequence of these limitations, no rates of treated or untreated specific psychiatric disorders were available in the United States that could be used to resolve issues of scientific and public policy concern in the 1970s. This gap was to be a major issue in the agenda of the President's Commission on Mental Health (1978) convened by President Carter upon taking office in 1977 (Carter, 1977).

The new paradigm

This revival of interest in psychopathology in the 1970s followed decades during which issues of diagnosis and classification had been held in low regard within the US mental health professions. Clinically, if the preferred treatment was individual psychotherapy, usually based on psychoanalysis, it mattered little what diagnostic category the patient was assigned to, because the treatment was directed not at an 'illness' but at the individual's personal conflicts and intrapsychic structures, such as ego functioning. Epidemiologically, indices of mental disability along a global mental-health–mental-illness continuum were used as the major measure of psychopathology. In this paradigm, the concepts and practices of traditional psychiatric diagnosis were in disrepute, criticised both on theoretical grounds and empirically because of low reliability in clinical practice and research studies.

The theoretical paradigm emphasising social and environmental factors (e.g. stress, urbanisation, and social class) and at the expense of biological factors (e.g. genetics) was thus dominant in clinical, research, and epidemiological endeavours. However, the profession of psychiatry came under attack from anti-psychiatrists, such as Szasz (1974) and Laing (1971); from social scientists, such as the labelling theorists and the anthropological relativists; and from lawyers, who applied the legal tactics of the civil rights movement to protect the rights of mental patients in institutions. The criticism of psychiatry during the 1960s included more than debates over issues of validity and reliability – it extended to the social and political criticism that psychiatry was serving as an agent of social control, disguising its power by benevolent rhetoric and the metaphor (or myth) of mental illness.

The current paradigm: strategies for validation of diagnostic classes

Confronted with these widespread and formidable criticisms, the US psychiatric research community responded slowly but vigorously in the 1970s. Gradually, a new paradigm evolved and was applied in studies of clinical diagnosis and treatment, and in genetics and epidemiology. The theoretical basis for the new paradigm was first articulated in England by Mayer-Gross *et al* (1954) in their influential but controversial textbook *Clinical Psychiatry*, and in the US by Robins & Guze (1970, 1972) and their associates at Washington University in St Louis.

As part of this paradigm shift, a validation strategy was formulated which has gained wide acceptance (Robins & Guze, 1972; Spitzer & Endicott, 1978). This strategy involved four major components:

(a) clinical description
(b) reliability
    (i) structured interviews
    (ii) operational criteria
    (iii) training
(c) validation
    (i) internal validity
    (ii) correlation with external domains
(d) testing aetiological hypotheses.

Firstly, the clinical syndrome is described with precision and standardisation by means of descriptive symptoms and manifest behaviour. The effort is made to remove inferences as to possible causation from the syndromal diagnostic criteria. This contamination of description and causation was a serious flaw in DSM–II (American Psychiatric Association, 1968). However, DSM–III attempted to be atheoretical with regard to the causes of individual disorders. It has been guided by a general theory of psychopathology and illness, but as regards the criteria of functional disorder for a specific disorder, aside from the organic disorders, the effort has been made to purge the diagnostic criteria of inferential causes or statements. Two exceptions to this rule are found in post-traumatic stress disorder and in adjustment disorder, in which the clinical symptoms are related to recent stressful events.

Having established the description of the syndrome, one then can test the extent to which different psychiatrists achieve reliability in making judgements as to appropriate assignment of the patient. These problems of reliability have been identified and their resolution attempted (Spitzer & Williams, 1980).

Thirdly, the establishment of the validity of a diagnostic category in general medicine or psychiatry requires the generation of evidence relevant to agreed criteria for what is a disease or a disorder. The assertion that schizophrenia is a 'disease' remains only a belief until appropriate evidence is generated. This involves the correlation of the syndrome with one or more external validators. The commonly agreed external validators are:

(a) clinical course and outcome
(b) response to treatment
(c) laboratory tests
(d) family and genetic studies
(e) epidemiological studies
(f) life events, personality and other psychological variables.

Validation and aetiology

The efforts at validation by operational criteria and correlation with external domain is not an end in itself but intended as part of a strategy to facilitate the testing of aetiological hypotheses. These aetiological hypotheses may refer to a presumed genetic cause, as in the case of bipolar disorder, or a presumed environmental cause, as with many personality disorders. Reliability and validity are intermediate achievements on the path of aetiological understanding. The problem, as observers such as Kendell (1988) pointed out, is that the existing symptom clusterings which result in the syndromes we are now attempting to validate in DSM–III and ICD–9 (World Health Organization, 1978) probably do not correspond to aetiological groupings.

The best example of this problem comes from genetic studies, which make the distinction between genotype and phenotype. It is likely that even in the case of a disorder, such as bipolar disorder, where the genetic evidence is increasingly strong, we probably will discover more than one genotype and the full phenotype range of expression of the genetic predisposition is probably not yet clear, although attempts to construct a concept of bipolar spectrum are an attempt to take cognisance of this likelihood and to arrange the symptom and phenomenological variables accordingly. Similarly, the concept of a schizophrenia spectrum postulates a genetically determined relationship between schizophrenia, schizoid personality and schizotypic personality disorder.

Conclusions

This chapter has traced the conceptual and historical development of thinking in the United States about diagnosis and classification, particularly developments since 1970 culminating in DSM–III and its revised edition. The 'paradigm' implicit in these strategies for reliability and validity has become widely accepted, at least among academic centres and research groups. It would be hard for a research project in psychopathology or clinical psychiatry to be funded by the NIMH if it did not include structured interviews and attention to issues of reliability and validity. These techniques have had a profound impact on related areas of research, notably genetic and family studies, epidemiological surveys, and follow-up studies of clinical course, outcome and therapeutic interventions, both psychopharmacological and psychotherapeutic. This is not to say that there have not been criticisms. There continues to be criticism, although less intense, from psychodynamic circles that the DSM–III system violates clinical experience and has contributed to a dehumanisation of psychiatry and to an enhanced status for biological psychiatry (Cooper & Michels, 1981; Fink, 1988; Klerman *et al*, 1984).

Although the categorical approach is dominant within psychiatric research centres, there continues to be active exploration of dimensional approaches by psychiatrists, particularly those concerned with personality disorders, and by psychologists and social scientists. To return to Kuhn's concept of progress and revolution in scientific fields, the new paradigm has become dominant and we are now in a period of what Kuhn would call 'normal science'. Numerous studies are underway on the reliability and validity of the multiple diagnostic categories developed and specified in DSM–II and DSM–III.

The planning for DSM–IV is underway and the early indications are that it will continue the basic structure of DSM–III. If Kuhn's predictions are correct, at some point the paradigm will encounter problems for which its approach is inadequate; there will be a period of puzzlement, the apparent consensus will break down, and at that point, a new paradigm may emerge.

References

AMERICAN PSYCHIATRIC ASSOCIATION (1968) *Diagnostic and Statistical Manual of Mental Disorders* (2nd edn) (DSM–II). Washington, DC: APA.
——— (1980) *Diagnostic and Statistical Manual of Mental Disorders* (3rd edn) (DSM–III). Washington, DC: APA.
CARTER, J. E. (1977) *Establishing a President's Commission on Mental Health.* Washington, DC: US Government Printing Office (executive order 11973).
COOPER, A., & MICHELS, R. (1981) Review of *Diagnostic and Statistical Manual of Mental Disorders* (Third Edition). *American Journal of Psychiatry*, **138**, 128–129.
FINK, P. J. (1988) Response to the Presidential address: Is "biopsychosocial" the psychiatric shibboleth? *American Journal of Psychiatry*, **145**, 1061–1067.
GLASS, A. J. (1958) Observations upon the epidemiology of mental illness in troops during warfare. In *Proceedings from the Symposium on Preventive and Social Psychiatry*, pp. 185–188. Washington, DC: National Research Council and Walter Reed Army Institution of Research.
GURIN, G. J., VEROOFF, J. & FELD, S. (1960) *Americans View their Mental Health: A Nationwide Interview Study.* New York: Basic Books.
HOLLINGSHEAD, A. B. & REDLICH, F. (1958) *Social Class and Mental Illness.* New York: Wiley.
KENDELL, R. E. (1988) What is a case? Food for thought for epidemiologists. *Archives of General Psychiatry*, **45**, 374–376.
KLERMAN, G. L. (1977) Mental illness, the medical model, and psychiatry. *Journal of Medicine and Philosophy*, **2**, 220–243.
——— (1978) The evolution of scientific nosology. In *Schizophrenia: Science and Practice* (ed. J. C. Shershow), pp. 99–121. Cambridge, MA: Harvard University Press.
——— (1986) Historical perspectives on contemporary schools of psychopathology. In *Contemporary Directions in Psychopathology Toward the DSM–IV* (eds T. Millon & G. L. Klerman), pp. 3–28. New York: Guilford Press.
——— (1989) Psychiatric diagnostic categories: issues of validity and measurement. *Journal of Health and Social Behavior*, **30**, 26–32.
——— (1990a) Paradigm shifts in USA psychiatric epidemiology since World War II. *Social Psychiatry and Psychiatric Epidemiology*, **25**, 27–32.
——— (1990b) The contemporary American scene: diagnosis and classification of mental disorders, alcoholism and drug abuse. In *Sources and Traditions of Classification in Psychiatry* (eds N. Sartorius, A. Jablensky, D. A. Regier, *et al*), pp. 99–139. New York: WHO and Hans Huber.
——— (1991) Comments on the Klerman–Stone Debate on Osheroff v. Chestnut Lodge (letter). *American Journal of Psychiatry*, **148**, 139–150.
———, VAILLANT, G., SPITZER, R., *et al* (1984) A debate on DSM–III. *American Journal of Psychiatry*, **141**, 539–553.

KUHN, T. S. (1970) *The Structure of Scientific Revolutions* (2nd edn). *International Encyclopedia of Unified Science*, vol. 2, no. 2. Chicago: University of Chicago Press.

LAING, R. D. (1971) *Psychiatry and Antipsychiatry*. New York: Harper and Row.

LANGNER, T. S. (1962) A 22 item screening score of psychiatric symptoms indicative of impairment. *Journal of Health and Human Behavior*, **3**, 269–276.

LEIGHTON, A., HARDING, J., MACKLIN, D. B., *et al* (1963) Psychiatric findings of the Stirling County Study. *American Journal of Psychiatry*, **119**, 1021–1031.

LORR, M. (1986) Classifying psychotics: dimensional and categorical approaches. In *Contemporary Directions in Psychopathology Toward the DSM–IV* (eds T. Millon & G. L. Klerman), pp. 331–346. New York: Guilford Press.

MAYER-GROSS, W., SLATER, E. & ROTH, M. (1954) *Clinical Psychiatry*. Baltimore: Williams and Wilkins.

MIROWSKY, J. & ROSS, C. E. (1989) Psychiatric diagnosis as reified measurement. *Journal of Health and Social Behavior*, **30**, 11–25.

MYERS, J. K. & BEAN, L. L. (1968) *A Decade Later: A Follow-Up of Social Class and Mental Illness*. New York: Wiley.

NATIONAL ADVISORY MENTAL HEALTH COUNCIL (1955) *Minutes and Proceedings. Public Health Service*. Washington, DC: US Government Printing Office.

PRESIDENT'S COMMISSION ON MENTAL HEALTH (1978) *Final Report*. Washington, DC: US Government Printing Office.

ROBINS, E. & GUZE, S. (1970) Establishment and psychiatric validity in psychiatric illness. Its application to schizophrenia. *American Journal of Psychiatry*, **126**, 983.

—— & —— (1972) Classification of affective disorders: the primary-secondary endogenous-reactive and neurotic-psychotic concepts. In *Psychobiology of Depressive Illness* (eds T. A. Williams, M. M. Katz & J. A. Shields, Jr), DHEW Publication Ho (HSM) 79-9053. Washington, DC: US Government Printing Office.

ROTHBLUM, E. D., SOLOMON, L. J. & ALBEE, G. W. (1986) A sociopolitical perspective of DSM–III. In *Contemporary Directions in Psychopathology Toward the DSM–IV* (eds T. Millon & G. L. Klerman), pp. 167–192. New York: Guilford Press.

SPITZER, R. L. & ENDICOTT, J. (1978) Medical and mental disorders: proposed definitions and criteria. In *Psychiatric Diagnosis* (eds R. L. Spitzer & D. F. Klein). New York: Raven Press.

—— & WILLIAMS, J. B. W. (1980) Classification of mental disorders. In *Comprehensive Textbook of Psychiatry* (eds H. I. Kaplan & J. Sadock), pp. 591–613. Baltimore: Williams and Wilkins.

SROLE, L., LANGNER, T. A., MICHAEL, S. T., *et al* (1962) *Mental Health in the Metropolis*. New York: McGraw-Hill.

STOUFFER, S. A., LUMSDAINE, A. A., LUMSDAINE, M. H., *et al* (1949) *The American Soldier: Combat and Its Aftermath*. Princeton, New Jersey: Princeton University Press.

SZASZ, T. (1974) *The Myth of Mental Illness*. New York: Harper and Row.

WEISSMAN, M. M. & KLERMAN, G. L. (1978) Epidemiology of mental disorders. *Archives of General Psychiatry*, **35**, 705–712.

—— & —— (1984) Epidemiology: purpose and historical overview. In *Social, Epidemiologic and Legal Psychiatry: A Textbook*, vol. 3 (ed. R. Michels), pp. 1–14. Philadelphia: J. B. Lippincott.

——, MYERS, J. K. & ROSS, C. (eds) (1987) *Community Surveys*. New Brunswick: Rutgers University Press.

WORLD HEALTH ORGANIZATION (1978) *Mental Disorders: Glossary and Guide to their Classification in Accordance with the Ninth Revision of the International Classification of Diseases* (ICD-9). Geneva: WHO.

7 A European perspective on the conceptual approaches to psychopathology

ERIK STRÖMGREN

This chapter chiefly examines the empirical, clinical observations which can be mentioned in support of the counterclaims over the nature of the functional psychoses. First, however, it is worth considering the different ways in which mental disorders can be at all similar, or dissimilar. They can be compared with regard to aetiology, to symptoms, to course, and to treatment response. These elements can be influenced by genetic and environmental factors. The genetic factors can be divided into specific factors and the non-specific gene environment, in the sense that the former may be a necessary condition for the occurrence of the disorder whereas the other genes can influence the vulnerability and, in addition, the clinical symptoms and the course, as can also the non-genetic environment. This implies that similarities between disorders need not be indicative of aetiological relationships.

As a model, the concept of constitutional types – as described by Kretschmer and his associates – can serve. According to this concept, certain affinities exist between special body and personality types and the liability to the different functional psychoses: schizophrenia was thought more likely to occur in leptosomatic persons with schizoid personality; manic–depressive disorder, in contrast, was considered more likely to originate in persons of pyknic body build and syntonic personality. Exceptions did, however, occur, and when they did this modified the clinical picture. For example, if schizophrenia arose in a pyknic person both the course and the symptoms would be more benign than in classic schizophrenia; in contrast, manic–depressive disorders in schizoid leptosomatic persons would have a more serious clinical picture, with delusions and hallucinations (Mauz, 1930). Similarly, the age of onset could greatly influence the clinical picture, for example giving nearly any psychosis arising in puberty a schizophreniform taint.

Such a system is not of course incompatible with the existence of different nosological entities, for example schizophrenia and manic–depressive disorder. The diversity in clinical pictures could be attributed solely to pathoplastic influences of different kinds and have nothing to do with supposed differences in aetiology. Nevertheless, it had to be taken into consideration that well known aetiologies of clearly different kinds could create clinical pictures indistinguishable from ordinary schizophrenia, such as Huntington's chorea, different intoxications, amphetamine psychosis, marijuana psychosis, etc.; at the other end of the scale of causative agents, delusional schizophrenia-like psychoses can arise as the result of mental conflicts, like Kretschmer's sensitive delusion of reference. Would it therefore be reasonable to talk only of a schizophrenic 'reaction type' which can be released by a number of agents? This would leave a great number of cases in which aetiology is unknown and which would, until we know better, just be called 'schizophrenic'. One could think similarly of an affective 'reaction type'.

The topic, our concepts of mental disorder, is closely connected with the old German idea of a unitary psychosis, '*Einheitspsychose*'. This term is traditionally connected with the name of Ernst Albert von Zeller (1804–77), who was especially influential during the 1830s and '40s. As a young man he was very impressed by the teachings of the philosopher Schleiermacher as a representative of the then prevailing Romantic school, which stressed the 'unity' of human life. Man was regarded as a psychosomatic unity and to make a distinction between mental and physical influences was not fashionable. Zeller regarded mental disorders as reactions to stress that caused a 'pathological irritation', especially of the abdominal neural ganglia and secondarily of the brain. Zeller's extensive psychiatric experience, especially in the psychiatric hospital at Winnenthal, near Stuttgart, gave him the impression that there was only one mental disease, but which could manifest itself in very different clinical forms, the course and sequence of which seemed to him to be quite unpredictable. He could distinguish only one general principle, namely that the first and most important symptom was melancholia, which was supposed to occur in all mental disorders, at least initially.

Wilhelm Griesinger was a pupil of Zeller at Winnenthal. He wrote the first truly realistic textbook of psychiatry, which appeared in 1845 and became a classic. Griesinger adhered to Zeller's theory of *Einheitspsychose* but stressed that all mental disorders must first have their basis in the brain. He gave a very realistic description of the different forms of mental disorders and he began to see the difference between those disorders that were caused by recognisable organic disorder of the brain and the other psychoses, which could be called 'functional'. The rapid progress of neuropathology which took place around the middle of the 19th century made this distinction even more meaningful. However, the greater part of the psychoses could not be demonstrated to have a definite morphological background, although most psychiatrists presumed its existence.

The inability of neuropathology to ascertain this foundation for the functional psychoses encouraged Kraepelin to try other methods of distinguishing the different psychoses, for example by correlating symptoms with course. Although his primary aim was a modest one, namely to establish practically useful correlations between symptoms and course, he also hoped in this way to distinguish between different nosological entities. His success was great and, in spite of all the criticism that has been uttered against his basic formulations and all the modifications which, among others, he himself also introduced in later years, there are some basic observations of Kraepelin's which are still fundamental to the thinking of most psychiatrists.

It should not be forgotten that shortly after Kraepelin's dichotomy of the psychoses had been generally recognised or at least well known, Karl Bonhoeffer (1909) made a quite different contribution to clinical psychiatry which has turned out to be of lasting value. Bonhoeffer, being especially interested in the different forms of organic psychoses, realised that the correlation between the specific aetiology and the symptoms and course in these cases was very loose. It became obvious to him that there was a thing like an organic reaction type which occurred in the great majority of cases in which a well known brain disorder was the basis for the symptoms. He convincingly described the acute and chronic organic reaction types, calling them exogenous reaction types.

The great sceptic in German psychiatry, Alfred Hoche (1912), was also a sharp opponent to Kraepelin's system, urging that in psychiatry one could only distinguish between different symptom clusters and syndromes, and that these distinctions could not in any way lead to the ascertainment of different nosological entities. But Kraepelin's teachings prevailed in Continental European psychiatry, where other schools also had an impact, initially that founded by Karl Kleist and later elaborated upon by Karl Leonhard. They tried to delimit different kinds of psychoses (episodic confusions, cycloid psychoses, etc.) which were supposed to be different from the two major Kraepelinian psychoses. Kleist tried to correlate these syndromes to localised disorders within the brain, whereas Leonhard became more interested in trying to find a specific genetic background for each of them, gradually subdividing the psychoses into many different forms which were regarded as separate nosological entities.

In the USA, the trend during the first half of the 19th century was of a very different kind, being dominated by the teaching of Adolf Meyer, whose basic viewpoint was definitely anti-nosological, regarding each patient as unique and each case history as originating as a result of numerous different kinds of agents and circumstances.

In the northern countries of Europe the situation has had, during most of the 20th century, some special characteristics with regard to the classification of the major psychoses (Bech, 1990). Under the influence of Karl Jaspers (1913) and the Danish psychiatrist August Wimmer (1916) it has been maintained that in addition to the two classic Kraepelinian psychoses there is a third important group of psychoses, namely the psychogenic or reactive psychoses. With regard to aetiology, genetic background, clinical features and course, this group is claimed to differ from both schizophrenia and manic–depressive disorder. Longitudinal studies performed over decades have confirmed the differences and genetic studies have shown their independence from the other major psychoses (Welner & Strömgren, 1958; Labhardt, 1963; McCabe, 1975; Bergman, 1976).

One further feature of Scandinavian psychiatry should be mentioned: the concept of schizophrenia has always been used in a relatively narrow sense. In particular, the so-called schizoaffective psychoses have been regarded as a group which in general is quite different from schizophrenia – although included in schizophrenia in ICD–8 and ICD–9 (World Health Organization, 1967, 1978); most of these cases have been regarded as variants of manic–depressive disorder, with which they seem to have more in common with regard to course and treatment response than they have with schizophrenia. There is thus no doubt that some cases which outside Scandinavia would be included in schizophrenia are in Scandinavia counted as either atypical manic–depressive disorders or reactive psychosis. This is, of course, of great importance when genetic studies from the different countries are compared, and is probably an explanation for the diversity of findings. The Scandinavian classification seems to fit the theory of genetic 'breeding true' better than do many studies from countries in which there is a wider concept of 'schizophrenia' and where the diagnosis of reactive psychosis is not generally made.

It may be useful to discuss in more detail findings which seem to contradict Kraepelin's dichotomy and support the idea of unitary psychosis. These findings fall mainly into three groups:

(a) the occurrence of mixed cases which seem to have symptoms from both Kraepelinian groups – schizoaffective disorders and the like

(b) apparent transition over time from manic–depressive symptoms to a schizophrenic clinical picture and course

(c) the occurrence in the same families of different forms of psychoses, schizophrenic and manic–depressive disorders occurring in the same sibship and, especially, children of manic–depressive parents being schizophrenic.

Each of these types of findings is discussed separately.

(a) Occurrence of different kinds of diagnoses among the members of the same family depends to a certain degree on the accuracy with which the symptoms are described. Some publications give the impression that as soon as delusions occur there is a tendency to suspect schizophrenia. Manic–depressives do of course often have true delusions, but on closer observation the general trend is that the delusions all rest, in the case of depression, on the feeling of guilt and the tendency to self-blame. Superficial description can claim that patients have ideas of persecution and are thus suspect for schizophrenia whereas, in fact, depressed patients do not actually *experience* persecution but feel they *deserve* persecution. Likewise with hallucinations: many depressives are said to hear voices, although the fact is that when they say that people are saying unfavourable things about them it is not something which they *hear*, they are just convinced that people must be talking unfavourably about them because they are 'bad'. If cases like these are described and analysed adequately it greatly reduces the number of schizoaffective cases, suspected as being true schizophrenia.

(b) With regard to the development of manic–depressive disorders into schizophrenic end-states, there has been a peculiar trend over time. During the first third of the 20th century such cases were often described and regarded as an important entity. In Continental and northern Europe such cases were often called '*Urstein psychoses*', named after a Polish psychiatrist Maurycy Urstein, who wrote two huge books about such cases (Urstein, 1909, 1912) which received much attention at that time. Urstein was strongly opposed to Kraepelin and was eager to show that there was no natural division between the two psychosis types described by Kraepelin. The title of his second book indicates his basic viewpoint: *Manisch–depressives und periodisches Irresein als Erscheinungsform der Katatonie* – manic–depressive and periodic mental disorder as manifestation of catatonia. He was convinced that there was just one kind of functional psychosis which could, however, show itself in many different forms. Urstein's books are full of case histories. He travelled a lot, especially in German-speaking countries, and collected case histories. It is not easy to see after which system he collected such histories, but he claimed to have seen some 1000 cases. Although there is doubt about the representativeness of his material, he succeeded in describing a number of cases which started with pure manic–depressive symptoms and ended in a state which could be called 'catatonic'.

Urstein psychosis was a well known term at the beginning of this century. When I first started working in psychiatric clinics in 1930 the term was familiar to everybody and we saw a considerable number of such cases. How can it be that these cases have nearly disappeared and the term *Urstein psychosis* likewise? Unfortunately there seems to have been nothing written about this disappearance of an impressive syndrome. To me the explanation is clear: when shock treatments were introduced they were often applied to just such patients, who responded miraculously to the treatment, and no symptoms were left which could be interpreted as schizophrenic symptoms. The conclusion must be that these patients really had manic–depressive psychoses with a malignant course and were subject to custodial maltreatment, given too many sedatives and hypnotics, disturbed, violent and noisy as they were, malignant developments which should now not be allowed and in most places do not develop.

(c) The apparent simultaneous occurrence of different types of psychoses in the same family is significantly reduced if reactive psychoses are treated separately. If this is done there is very little overlap. There are, however, important exceptions, by far the most important being the peculiar and much discussed observation that whereas it seems that a schizophrenic person has never had manic–depressive children, the opposite is not infrequent. If these two observations are true, it seems to be impossible to give a genetic explanation for them. On the one hand, they are, on face value, incompatible with the dichotomy hypothesis but on the other they are, paradoxically, also incompatible with the continuum hypothesis. A very thorough analysis of all relevant observations of this kind should be the first step before any conclusions are made.

One fact is striking: these so-called 'schizophrenic' children of manic–depressive parents have all had psychoses which started early, mostly in puberty. It is well known that any psychosis, regardless of aetiology, which arises in puberty can acquire schizophrenic symptoms, and then ultimately turn out to be a non-schizophrenic disorder. There is no doubt that some of the cases can be explained in this way.

A more systematic study has been published by Taschev & Roglev (1976). They studied 210 families comprising 441 psychotic patients. The 109 psychotic parents had 117 psychotic children. There was great similarity between the psychoses of parents and children. Some parents and children differed with regard to clinical diagnosis, but even then the clinical pictures were in fact similar. A general trend was that the psychoses in the children started early. This is probably mainly a selective artefact, since at this stage the children with early onset would have greater chance of being recorded as 'cases', so there is as yet no need for a theory of 'anteposition'. It can be concluded that even in this large collection of data, there is no clear-cut case of manic–depressive disorder in the parent and schizophrenia in the child.

Some further important findings should be mentioned. As yet no case has been published in which one homozygotic twin has been schizophrenic and the other manic–depressive. Moreover, studies of offspring of two psychotics have shown that if one parent is manic–depressive and the other schizophrenic, the two disorders segregate in the offspring. This would be difficult to explain on the basis of the continuum hypothesis.

It may be concluded that there is no strong empirical evidence against the dichotomy along Kraepelinian lines if the existence of a few additional nosological entities is taken into consideration. But this is, of course, not a proof, only a suggestion that the dichotomy is still, in general, a valid hypothesis.

From a research viewpoint it must be stressed that for the performance of these delicate clinical and genetic studies, instruments like those contained in the World Health Organization's *International Classification of Diseases*, the American Psychiatric Association's *Diagnostic and Statistical Manual of Mental*

Disorders (DSM), or the other diagnostic systems such as the Research Diagnostic Criteria (RDC) of Spitzer *et al* (1978), are too crude; they cannot delimit natural, not to say nosological entities, which anyway was not the intention or ambition behind their construction. From the Scandinavian viewpoint it is a serious defect in DSM and RDC that there is no natural place for reactive psychoses, which type of disorder therefore occurs as an inadequate admixture of other natural groups. This is dangerous, not only for the treatment of these patients but also for the validity of research performed by means of these techniques.

References

BECH, P. (1990) Diagnostic and classification tradition of mental disorders in the 20th century in Scandinavia. In *Sources and Traditions of Classification in Psychiatry* (eds N. Sartorius, A. Jablensky, *et al*). Toronto: Hogrefe & Huber.
BERGMAN, W. (1976) *Om Psykogena Psykoser av Konfusionstyp. En Efterundersökning av 143 Patienter.* Stockholm: Karolinska Institutets psykiatriska klinik vid S:t Görans sjukhus.
BONHOEFFER, K. (1909) Zur Frage der exogenen Psychosen. *Zentralblatt für Nervenheilkunde und Psychiatrie*, **32**, 499–505.
GRIESINGER, W. (1845) *Pathologie und Therapie der psychischen Krankheiten für Ärzte und Studierende.* Stuttgart: Adolph Krabbe.
HOCHE, A. (1912) Die Bedetung der Symptomenkomplexe in der Psychiatrie. *Zentralblatt für die gesamte Neurologie und Psychiatrie*, **5**, 804–810.
JASPERS, K. (1913) Allgemeine Psychopathologie. *Ein Leitfaden für Studierende, Ärzte und Psychologen.* Berlin: Springer.
LABHARDT, F. (1963) *Die schizophrenieähnlichen Emotionspsychosen. Ein Beitrag zur Abgrenzung schizophrenieartiger Zustandsbilder.* Berlin: Springer.
MAUZ, F. (1930) *Die Prognostik der endogenen Psychosen.* Leipzig: Georg Thieme.
MCCABE, M. S. (1975) Reactive psychoses. A clinical and genetic investigation. *Acta Psychiatrica Scandinavica* (suppl. 259).
SPITZER, R. L., ENDICOTT, J. & ROBINS, E. (1978) *Research Diagnostic Criteria (RDC) for a Selected Group of Functional Disorders* (3rd edn). New York: New York State Psychiatric Institute.
TASCHEV, T. & ROGLEV, M. (1976) Vergleichende Untersuchungen an Psychosen von Eltern, Kindern und Geschwistern. *Archiv für Psychiatrie und Nervenkrankheiten*, **222**, 377–386.
URSTEIN, M. (1909) *Die Dementia praecox und ihre Stellung zum manisch-depressiven Irresein.* Berlin, Wien: Urban & Schwarzenberg.
—— (1912) *Manisch-depressives und periodisches Irresein als Erscheinungsform der Katatonie.* Berlin: Urban & Schwarzenberg.
WELNER, J. & STRÖMGREN, E. (1958) Clinical and genetic studies on benign schizophreniform psychoses based on a follow-up. *Acta Psychiatrica Scandinavica*, **33**, 377–399.
WIMMER, A. (1916) Psykogene Sindssygdomsformer. In *St Hans Hospital 1816–1915* (ed. A. Wimmer), pp. 85–216. København: Gad.
WORLD HEALTH ORGANIZATION (1967) *Manual of the International Statistical Classification of Diseases, Injuries, and Causes of Death, 1965 revision* (8th edn) (ICD–8). Geneva: WHO.
—— (1978) *Mental Disorders: Glossary and Guide to their Classification in Accordance with the Ninth Revision of the International Classification of Diseases* (ICD–9). Geneva: WHO.

8 Unitary psychosis and the psychiatry of old age

DAVID KAY

A unitary theory of the functional psychoses would account *inter alia* for the failure to demonstrate a dichotomy between the two major prototypes (Kendell & Brockington, 1980). As described in the preceding chapters, the position of schizoaffective psychosis is pivotal to this question, since it could constitute the bridge between affective psychosis and schizophrenia (Crow, 1986).

Longitudinal studies

The psychiatry of old age could contribute to our knowledge in various ways. The panoramic view of past life obtained from the vantage-point of old age should help to assess the stability of syndromes over time and reveal the continuity or otherwise of the major groups into old age. Those with psychotic syndromes should have recovered from their adolescent turmoil and the syndromes have revealed their true identities. Intermediate forms may be found to have merged into one or other of the major types or have remained distinct.

Unfortunately, geriatric psychiatry has contributed little to this particular question. However, long-term follow-up studies of functional psychoses show that both psychopathologically and in social functioning the outcome in schizoaffective psychosis is intermediate between the major forms (Harrow & Grossman, 1984; Angst, 1986; Gross *et al*, 1986; Marneros *et al*, 1986a,b). Relatively more schizoaffective psychoses compared with schizophrenia have a full remission and relatively fewer end in a defect state.

There appears to be considerable interchange between one group and another. This should be seen against the background of diagnostic change between schizophrenia and affective psychosis in about 10% of cases over a long period (Sheldrick *et al*, 1977; Angst, 1986). Marneros *et al* (1986a) found that 39% of schizoaffective cases remained stable while 61% were 'polymorphous' with later pure schizophrenic or pure affective episodes. However, nearly all cases had at least one further episode with concurrent schizophrenic and affective syndromes and most sequential cases became concurrent during their course (Marneros *et al*, 1986*a*).

Remitting psychoses of all types are associated with a decrease in psychotic symptoms (delusions and hallucinations) in later episodes (Winokur *et al*, 1985), schizoaffective psychosis being intermediate between schizophrenia and affective psychosis in this respect; however, it was characterised by a larger number of episodes and hospital admissions than the other psychoses and the symptoms over the first ten episodes at least remained virtually identical to those in the index admission. Since the course of schizophrenia is usually chronic rather than episodic, the outcome in schizoaffective psychosis could be regarded as intermediate in severity between the two other major psychoses.

Clinical studies of late-life psychoses

European studies

Schizoaffective psychosis is said rarely to begin after the age of 30. Only Post (1971) seems to have studied late-life schizoaffective psychosis as such. In two earlier monographs (Post, 1962, 1966) schizophrenic features – paranoid delusions and "bizarre schizophreniform symptoms" – were found in 38% of patients with affective illnesses; in 3% the illness developed into schizophrenia. In patients with persistent persecutory ideas affective symptoms were found in 58% and in 22% were "at times severe and dominated the clinical picture"; 16% had a history of episodes of depression, although only 3% had needed treatment.

Janzarik (1957) had already reported observations on 50 elderly schizophrenics who had fallen ill after age 60. Post (1966), quoting Janzarik, remarked that there was often difficulty in excluding affective illnesses with paranoid symptoms and that Janzarik had regretted the passing of the unitary concept of psychosis.

In 1971 Post described 29 patients with schizoaffective disorder. These had shown simultaneously or in succession schizophrenic and affective symptoms and had remained ill for long periods. The mood changes were the most prominent feature. In many ways the symptoms were intermediate between those of the affective and paranoid groups studied during the same period. Examples of all three types of psychosis occurred in the families. As regards treatment, changes from one category of drug to another were frequent and the outcome disappointing.

Roth (1987) pointed out that depressive symptoms rarely caused difficulties in diagnosis of late paraphrenia, since the scope of paranoid symptoms extended well beyond themes consistent with a diagnosis of affective psychosis. However, a small minority of cases began with affective psychosis with unusually pronounced and wide-ranging paranoid hallucinatory features which dominated the picture in later episodes. Holden (1987) reported that after a ten-year follow-up, five of 24 cases (20%) of late paraphrenia could be diagnosed as schizoaffective psychosis. This was on the basis of at least one subsequent affective episode. These patients were characterised by auditory hallucinations and a good response to treatment. It is interesting that an equal number of the original group with functional paranoid psychoses had been excluded because review of the initial presentation suggested they were suffering from affective psychosis with holothymic (mood-congruent) paranoid delusions.

North American studies: DSM–III criteria

The restriction of the diagnosis of schizophrenia in DSM–III (American Psychiatric Association, 1980) to cases beginning before age 45 years stimulated inquiries into the existence of functional psychoses of late onset. These appear to have confirmed the European findings in most respects (Rabins *et al*, 1984, 1987*a*; Craig & Bregman, 1988; Jeste *et al*, 1988*a*; Pearlson & Rabins, 1988): cases with onset after 45 years who fulfilled DSM–III criteria for schizophrenia or schizophreniform disorder (apart from age) did exist and responded well to neuroleptic drugs. However, a small proportion fulfilled criteria for delusional disorder.

Some patients with DSM–III mood disorder were found to have delusions, hallucinations and first-rank symptoms and it was possible that some of these might really have been schizophrenics. In one study, 20% of the schizophrenics later developed prominent mood disorders (Craig & Bregman, 1988). The existence of an intermediate group corresponding to schizoaffective disorder is not discussed in any detail in these studies because attention was focused on schizophrenia.

Leuchter & Spar (1985) started with patients with psychotic symptoms (delusions and hallucinations) arising for the first time after 65 years of age, irrespective of diagnosis, and found more patients with major mood disorder (36%) than with paranoid disorder or schizophrenia (21%). In the remaining 43% the diagnosis was organic mental disorder. They noted many changes of diagnosis between the functional groups, more than between these and the organic groups, and suggested that the distinction between mood disorder and schizophrenia could be difficult to make. This could have been due to insufficiently clear criteria or to a real lack of a precise boundary.

Mood-incongruent features and diagnostic problems

If, as has been reported (Baldwin, 1988), psychotic and non-psychotic affective disorders differ from each other in response to treatment and in outcome, late-onset schizophrenia should only be compared with other late-life psychoses, as opposed to other disorders, although this has not been systematically done.

In Europe schizophrenic symptoms usually have priority over mood symptoms. For instance, in Crow's (1986) continuum model, mood-incongruent delusions are placed towards the schizophrenic end. But in DSM-III, major depression is compatible with delusions and hallucinations provided that prominent mood symptoms are also present. An important point is that the delusions and hallucinations may be mood-incongruent. Hence, patients with mood-incongruent features would be schizophrenic in Europe but mood disordered in North America. This may partly account for the smaller proportion of late-onset psychotic patients with schizophrenia and for the larger proportion with mood disorder in North American clinics.

Conclusions

It would seem that a forced choice of one or other of the two major groups can be made without great difficulty in the large majority of cases. However, there is considerable overlap in symptoms and when diagnostic rules are relaxed a much larger intermediate group can be constructed. The complexity of the diagnostic criteria for schizoaffective psychosis in DSM-III-R (American Psychiatric Association, 1987) suggests that there is a real difficulty in defining its boundaries. For instance, Angst (1986) categorised 31% of a series of 709 patients with functional psychoses as schizoaffective, while in the Cologne study, where both a schizophrenic *and* a melancholic or manic syndrome had to be present concurrently or sequentially, the proportion of schizoaffective diagnoses was about 7% of all schizophrenic and suspected schizophrenic cases (Marneros *et al*, 1986*b*).

Separating the prototypic psychoses from each other and from schizo-affective psychosis poses very similar problems in the late-onset and early-onset psychoses. The range of symptoms suggests that a late-onset schizoaffective group could be defined so as to be large or small. However, a full schizophrenic and affective syndrome equivalent to major depression (or mania) concurrently or sequentially, should be required, including the DSM-III fifth-digit code for psychotic features, for comparison with schizo-phrenic and affective psychosis. Data for late-life psychoses are scanty and further inquiries are called for. Recognition of the syndrome of late paraphrenia facilitated inquiry and demonstrated the efficacy of neuroleptic treatment. Post (1971) considered that provisional recognition of schizoaffective psychosis might also lead to improved understanding and treatment.

Late-onset psychosis and organic brain disease

An organic cause for at least some cases of late-onset psychoses was always an important issue (Kay & Roth, 1961). When patients presenting with affective or schizophrenic disorders *without* psycho-organic symptoms were followed up there appeared to be no definite increase either in the later incidence of organic brain disease or in mortality (Roth, 1956; Post, 1962, 1966). However, psychological assessment was usually limited to simple clinical tests and neuropathology was not studied. It was established, however, that typical functional syndromes indistinguishable in form and content from those seen in patients with normal brains could occur in the presence of brain disease and that specific organic or symptomatic syndromes could not be clinically separated from the remainder, until they declared their presence during the course of illness (Post, 1966; Shulman & Post, 1980).

Neuroimaging offered a fresh approach, and these studies are examined below, with the unitary concept still in mind, comparing the incidence and significance of structural brain abnormalities in late-onset psychoses of schizophrenic and affective type (but studies seldom distinguish psychotic from non-psychotic affective disorders). No imaging study of late-onset schizoaffective psychosis has been reported.

The neuroimaging studies

Ventricular enlargement

Computerised tomography scans were studied in elderly affective patients by Jacoby & Levy (1980) and brain density measured (in Hounsfield units) by Jacoby *et al* (1983). Patients with late paraphrenia were studied by Naguib & Levy (1987) and by Rabins *et al* (1987*b*). In both groups the ventricle : brain ratio (VBR) was less than occurs in Alzheimer's disease and in late paraphrenia it was increased compared with that in age-matched controls. Brain density in depressives was between that of the demented and controls (Jacoby *et al*, 1983). The normal pattern of correlations between VBR, cortical atrophy and age was disturbed in both groups. A subgroup of depressives with enlarged ventricles and decreased brain density was identified whose depression began after the age of 60; two-year mortality was significantly raised only in this subgroup, but there was no evidence that they were misdiagnosed cases of dementia (Jacoby *et al*, 1981). In late paraphrenia no subgroup was apparent; the VBR showed no relation to duration of illness, and generalised cortical atrophy was absent; mortality was not increased (Hymas *et al*, 1989).

The interpretation of the findings was different. Structural change in the brain causing ventricular enlargement rather than age-related cortical atrophy was considered the probable basis of late paraphrenia (Burns *et al*, 1989). In depression the onset in late life was thought to be related to the ageing process (Jacoby *et al*, 1981).

White-matter lesions

Jacoby & Levy (1980) found evidence of cerebrovascular disease in 12% of elderly affectives compared with 2% of age-matched controls; it was occult in 5%. Miller & Lesser (1988) and Miller *et al* (1989) found occult white-matter lesions, frontal or subfrontal, in a proportion of elderly patients with late-onset psychoses resembling schizophrenia, in the absence of dementia or clinical signs of neurological disease. Comparable lesions were not found in healthy age-matched controls. Clinically, there were complex delusions, with or without hallucinations, associated with abnormal behaviour and evidence of frontal lobe dysfunction (Miller *et al*, 1989). A disconnection syndrome was postulated.

Coffey *et al* (1989), using magnetic resonance imaging (MRI), reported white-matter hyperintensities, representing periventricular translucencies (leucoencephalopathy, araiosis), in 100% of elderly depressives referred for electroconvulsive therapy (ECT). The white-matter hyperintensities were more severe than similar areas seen in a smaller proportion of controls and were associated with gross structural brain changes, such as cortical atrophy (in 96%) and enlargement of the lateral ventricle (in 69%). Clinically, the depression was usually of late onset and resistant to antidepressants, and in 30% was of psychotic type. It was postulated that structural brain lesions may interact with ageing to bring about depression. However, MRI reveals white-matter lesions in 20–30% of clinically healthy subjects and their pathology and clinical significance is often uncertain (Kirkpatrick & Hayman, 1987).

Neuropsychological findings

Both elderly affective (Jacoby & Levy, 1980) and late paraphrenic (Naguib & Levy, 1987) patients were found to be cognitively impaired compared with age-matched controls. There was no evidence in these studies of a specific cerebral basis since there was no correlation with CT measures in either group. The cognitive impairment in depressives was attributed to pseudodementia. However, Pearlson *et al* (1989*a*) found that patients showing the dementia syndrome of depression (pseudodementia) but not other depressed patients differed significantly in VBR and CT density scores from normal controls. Although the values approximated to those of patients with probable Alzheimer's disease, follow-up did not suggest that either subgroup was in the early stages of progressive dementia. This was also the conclusion in a three- to four-year follow-up of the patients with late paraphrenia.

However, Holden (1987) had reported that a subgroup of patients with late paraphrenia with initial poor cognition became overtly demented after two years. An organic substrate was postulated in late paraphrenia (Hymas *et al*, 1989) and underlying structural abnormalities of unknown kind in depression (Pearlson *et al*, 1989*a*). The frontal lobe deficits found by Miller *et al* (1989) in their patients with late-onset psychoses were apparently newly acquired.

Involuntary movements

The presence of involuntary movements (tardive dyskinesia) in elderly schizophrenic patients may be due to disease factors and age rather than use of neuroleptics. There appears to be a consistent relationship between the presence of involuntary movements, cognitive impairment and negative symptoms, which is found not only in chronic schizophrenics but also in bipolar patients (Waddington *et al*, 1989).

Conclusions

The similarities in neuroimaging and neuropsychological findings between late-onset affective and schizophrenic psychoses are striking. An increased VBR and the presence of white-matter hyperintensities have been reported in both disorders, together with some degree of cognitive impairment in a proportion of cases. However, over the short term, at least, dementia seldom develops. In affective psychosis the increase in VBR has been interpreted as further evidence for a non-specific effect of brain ageing (Jacoby & Levy, 1980). A similar change in late paraphrenia has been related to a pre-existing structural lesion, constituting a non-specific risk factor (Pearlson & Rabins, 1988; Burns *et al*, 1989). However, it is possible that the structural changes in affective psychosis also are life-long (Pearlson *et al*, 1989*a*). Poor performance on neuropsychological tests could also be due to life-long factors.

Occult, clinically unsuspected white-matter lesions revealed by neuro-imaging appear to be an aetiological factor in some cases of either type of psychosis. The occurrence of these lesions is age-related and they may be commoner in late-onset than in early-onset psychoses. Their numerical significance is uncertain; no coarse brain disease was found in a series of 29 patients with late-onset schizophrenia (over age 45 years) who underwent CT scans (Rabins *et al*, 1987*b*).

Psychosis and brain disease in younger patients

The recent findings in late-onset psychoses at first sight suggest that these psychoses are secondary to brain disease and differ in some fundamental way from those of earlier onset. However, the last decade has seen growing evidence for the existence and significance of brain changes in schizophrenia (Weinberger, 1987; Reynolds, 1989; Lantos, 1988; Lewis, 1989). The changes are not secondary to treatment, are not correlated with duration of illness, and seem not to increase with passage of time; according to a developmental model they are acquired early in life and may be non-specific. The lesion reveals its presence in dramatic fashion only when certain areas of brain become functionally active (Weinberger, 1987). The cognitive deficits that have been demonstrated in schizophrenia (Johnstone *et al*, 1978; Taylor & Abrams, 1984) could be related to the presence of life-long structural change.

The developmental model refers only to schizophrenia. But when VBRs in affective psychosis and schizophrenia have been measured in the same study and compared with each other, the results are usually similar and both differ from controls (Owens *et al*, 1985; Pearlson *et al*, 1985), although ventricular enlargement is present in only a minority of cases of either type. Harvey *et al* (1990) and Rieder *et al* (1983) found that the mean VBRs and sulcal ratings of patients with schizophrenia, affective psychosis or schizoaffective psychosis did not differ significantly from each other. Jeste *et al* (1988*b*) concluded that "in every area in which structural abnormalities have been found in neuroradiological studies of schizophrenia, abnormalities of similar magnitude have also been demonstrated in affective disorders".

At another level, the existence of organic disease presenting as functional psychosis has been known for years. Johnstone *et al* (1987) found 6% of first-episode schizophrenics had organic disease which could have contributed to the mental state. Neuroimaging studies may increase the proportion of such cases, which would be classifiable as organic delusional disorder in DSM–III–R. Such cases may occur at any age. Interest in structural change in affective psychosis has focused more on the site and laterality of gross brain disease when this is present, and the disorder may then be classified as secondary depression, mania or organic mood disorder (Shulman & Post, 1980; Cummings, 1986). As in schizophrenia, the underlying disease may not be clinically obvious. Limbic and basal ganglia lesions and disordered dopaminergic pathways may be involved in delusional disorders, while monoaminergic functions may be affected in secondary mania (Cummings, 1986). A feature of late-onset schizophrenia is the vivid hallucinosis in various modalities (Pearlson *et al*, 1989*b*), presumably an expression of the positive, type I, symptoms usually responsive to neuroleptics and possibly associated with dopaminergic overactivity (Weinberger, 1987). It remains to be shown how much commoner these organic psychoses are in later than in earlier life.

These studies bring the psychoses of later and earlier life closer together. The developmental model proposed for schizophrenia does not explain the late onset, but this is part of the wider problem of age of onset. The similarities between schizophrenia and affective psychosis are in keeping with the proposition that there is a "general biology of psychosis" (Freedman, 1975). Genetic factors are known to be present and it is possible that the similarities between these psychoses are a consequence of mutant alleles at one site, though it is unlikely that only two forms of endogenous psychosis exist. However, family studies do not support a separate schizoaffective gene (Zerbin-Rudin, 1986).

Conclusions

There is considerable overlap of schizophrenic and affective symptoms in the late-onset psychoses, but systematic studies are few and it is not clear how often the full syndromes of schizophrenia and affective psychosis as defined by modern diagnostic systems actually occur simultaneously or sequentially in the same patient.

Recent advances in brain imaging suggested a greater role for structural brain disease in late-life psychosis than previous studies had determined. However, organic components in the functional psychoses have become increasingly evident at all ages. Developmental models based on quantitative post-mortem and CT studies in schizophrenia and controls have proposed that structural change in the brain is present in early life, and they may be applicable to a proportion of cases with late onset although they do not explain the long delay. Similar models have not been proposed for affective or schizoaffective psychoses, but could be relevant for these psychoses. There are also cases in which gross brain lesions are revealed by neuroimaging, but their numerical importance in the aetiology of late-life psychosis remains to be determined.

Despite lack of data about late-life disorders, the relation between schizophrenic, schizoaffective and affective psychoses appears to be similar whatever the age of onset. The differences are difficult to interpret simply as a matter of severity. These psychoses appear, rather, to be biologically closely related disorders, susceptible to the same non-specific factors. Specific genetic factors seem to be present in schizophrenia and affective psychosis but there is at present little evidence for a separate schizoaffective gene.

References

AMERICAN PSYCHIATRIC ASSOCIATION (1980) *Diagnostic and Statistical Manual of Mental Disorders* (3rd edn) (DSM–III). Washington, DC: APA.
—— (1987) *Diagnostic and Statistical Manual of Mental Disorders* (3rd edn, revised) (DSM–III-R). Washington, DC: APA.
ANGST, J. (1986) The course of schizoaffective disorders. In *Schizoaffective Psychoses* (eds A. Marneros & M. T. Tsuang). Berlin: Springer.

BALDWIN, R. C. (1988) Delusional and non-delusional depression in late life: evidence for distinct types. *British Journal of Psychiatry*, **152**, 39–44.

BURNS, A., CARRICK, J., AMES, D., *et al* (1989) The cerebral cortical appearance in late paraphrenia. *International Journal of Geriatric Psychiatry*, **4**, 31–34.

COFFEY, C. E., FIGIEL, G. S., DJANG, W. T., *et al* (1989) White matter hyperintensity on magnetic resonance imaging: clinical and neuroanatomic correlates in the depressed elderly. *Journal of Neuropsychiatry*, **1**, 135–144.

CRAIG, T. J. & BREGMAN, Z. (1988) Late onset schizophrenia-like illness. *Journal of the American Geriatrics Society*, **36**, 104–107.

CROW, T. J. (1986) The continuum of psychosis and its implication for the structure of the gene. *British Journal of Psychiatry*, **149**, 419–429.

CUMMINGS, J. L. (1986) Organic psychoses. *Psychiatric Clinics of North America*, **9**, 293–311.

FREEDMAN, D. X. (1975) Biology of the major psychoses: a comparative analysis. *Research Publication; Association of Nervous and Mental Disorders*, **54**, vii–viii.

GROSS, G., HUBER, G. & ARMBRUSTER, B. (1986) Schizoaffective psychoses: long-term prognosis and symptomatology. In *Schizoaffective Psychoses* (eds A. Marneros & M. T. Tsuang). Berlin: Springer.

HARROW, M. & GROSSMAN, L. S. (1984) Outcome in schizoaffective disorder: a critical review and reevaluation of the literature. *Schizophrenia Bulletin*, **10**, 87–108.

HARVEY, I., WILLIAMS, M., TOONE, B. K., *et al* (1990) The ventricular-brain ratio (VBR) in functional psychoses: the relationship of lateral ventricular and total intracranial area. *Psychological Medicine*, **20**, 55–62.

HOLDEN, N. L. (1987) Late paraphrenia or the paraphrenias? A descriptive study with a 10-year follow-up. *British Journal of Psychiatry*, **150**, 635–639.

HYMAS, N., NAGUIB, M. & LEVY, R. (1989) Late paraphrenia – a follow-up study. *International Journal of Geriatric Psychiatry*, **4**, 23–29.

JACOBY, R. J. & LEVY, R. (1980) Computed tomography in the elderly. 3. Affective disorder. *British Journal of Psychiatry*, **136**, 270–275.

——, LEVY, R. & BIRD, J. M. (1981) Computed tomography and the outcome of affective disorder: a follow-up study of elderly patients. *British Journal of Psychiatry*, **139**, 288–292.

——, DOLAN, R. J., LEVY, R., *et al* (1983) Quantitative computed tomography in elderly depressed patients. *British Journal of Psychiatry*, **143**, 124–127.

JANZARIK, W. (1957) Zur Problematik schizophrener Psychoses im höherer Lebensalter. *Nervenarzt*, **28**, 535.

JESTE, D. V., HARRIS, M. J., PEARLSON, G. D., *et al* (1988*a*) Late-onset schizophrenia: studying clinical variability. *Psychiatric Clinics of North America*, **11**, 1–13.

——, LOHR, J. B. & GOODWIN, F. K. (1988*b*) Neuroanatomical studies of major affective disorders: a review and suggestions for further research. *British Journal of Psychiatry*, **153**, 444–459.

JOHNSTONE, E. C., CROW, T. J., FRITH, C. D., *et al* (1978) The dementia of dementia praecox. *Acta Psychiatrica Scandinavica*, **57**, 305–324.

——, MACMILLAN, J. F. & CROW, T. J. (1987) The occurrence of organic disease of possible or probable aetiological significance in a population of 268 cases of first episode schizophrenia. *Psychological Medicine*, **17**, 371–379.

KAY, D. W. K. & ROTH, M. (1961) Environmental and hereditary factors in the schizophrenias of old age (''late paraphrenia'') and their bearing on the general problem of causation in schizophrenia. *Journal of Mental Science*, **110**, 668–686.

KENDELL, R. E. & BROCKINGTON, I. F. (1980) The identification of disease entities and the relations between schizophrenia and affective psychoses. *British Journal of Psychiatry*, **137**, 324–331.

KIRKPATRICK, J. B. & HAYMAN, L. A. (1987) White-matter lesions in MR imaging of clinically healthy brains of elderly subjects: possible pathologic basis. *Radiology*, **162**, 509–511.

LANTOS, P. L. (1988) The neuropathology of schizophrenia: a critical review of recent work. In *Schizophrenia: The Major Issues* (eds P. Bebbington, P. McGuffin). London: Mental Health Foundation/Heinemann.

LEUCHTER, A. F. & SPAR, J. E. (1985) The late-onset psychoses: clinical and diagnostic features. *Journal of Nervous and Mental Diseases*, **173**, 488–494.

LEWIS, S. W. (1989) Congenital risk factors for schizophrenia. *Psychological Medicine*, **19**, 5–13.

MARNEROS, A. & TSUANG, M. T. (1986) Schizoaffective disorders: present level and future perspective. In *Schizoaffective Psychoses* (eds A. Marneros & M. T. Tsuang). Berlin: Springer.

——, ROHDE, A., DEISTER, A., *et al* (1986a) Schizoaffective psychoses: the prognostic value of the affective component. In *Schizoaffective Psychoses* (eds A. Marneros & M. T. Tsuang). Berlin: Springer.

——, DEISTER, A. & ROHDE, A. (1986b) The Cologne study on schizoaffective disorders and schizophrenia suspecta. In *Schizoaffective Psychoses* (eds A. Marneros & M. T. Tsuang). Berlin: Springer.

MILLER, B. L. & LESSER, I. M. (1988) Late-life psychosis and modern neuroimaging. *Psychiatric Clinics of North America*, **11**, 33–46.

——, LESSER, I. M., BOONE, K., *et al* (1989) Brain white-matter lesions and psychosis. *British Journal of Psychiatry*, **155**, 73–78.

NAGUIB, M. & LEVY, R. (1987) Late paraphrenia: neuropsychological impairment and structural brain abnormalities on computed tomography. *International Journal of Geriatric Psychiatry*, **2**, 83–90.

OWENS, D. G. C., JOHNSTONE, E. C., CROW, T. J., *et al* (1985) Lateral ventricular size in schizophrenia: relationship to the disease process and its clinical manifestations. *Psychological Medicine*, **15**, 27–42.

PEARLSON, G. D., GARBACZ, D. J., MOBERG, P. J., *et al* (1985) Symptomatic, familial, perinatal, and social correlates of computerized axial tomography (CAT) changes in schizophrenics and bipolars. *Journal of Nervous and Mental Diseases*, **173**, 42–50.

—— & RABINS, P. (1988) The late-onset psychoses: possible risk factors. *Psychiatric Clinics of North America*, **11**, 15–32.

——, ——, KIM, W. S., *et al* (1989a) Structural brain CT changes and cognitive deficits in elderly depressives with and without reversible dementia ('pseudodementia'). *Psychological Medicine*, **19**, 573–584.

——, KREGER, L., RABINS, P. V., *et al* (1989b) A chart review of late-onset and early-onset schizophrenia. *American Journal of Psychiatry*, **146**, 1568–1574.

POST, F. (1962) *The Significance of Affective Symptoms in Old Age*. Maudsley monograph no. 10. London: Oxford University Press.

—— (1966) *Persistent Persecutory States of the Elderly*. Oxford: Pergamon Press.

—— (1971) Schizo-affective symptomatology in late life. *British Journal of Psychiatry*, **118**, 437–445.

RABINS, P., PAUKER, S. & THOMAS, J. (1984) Can schizophrenia begin after age 44? *Comprehensive Psychiatry*, **25**, 290–293.

——, MCHUGH, P. R., PAUKER, S., *et al* (1987a) The clinical features of late onset schizophrenia. In *Schizophrenia and Aging* (eds N. Miller & G. Cohen), pp. 235–238. New York: Guilford Press.

——, PEARLSON, G. D., JAYARAM, G., *et al* (1987b) Increased ventricle-to-brain ratio in late onset schizophrenia. *American Journal of Psychiatry*, **144**, 1216–1218.

REYNOLDS, G. P. (1989) Beyond the dopamine hypothesis: the neurochemical pathology of schizophrenia. *British Journal of Psychiatry*, **155**, 305–316.

RIEDER, R. O., MANN, L. S., WEINBERGER, D. R., *et al* (1983) Computed tomographic scans in patients with schizophrenia, schizoaffective, and bipolar affective disorder. *Archives of General Psychiatry*, **40**, 735–739.

ROTH, M. (1956) The natural history of mental disorder in old age. *Journal of Mental Science*, **101**, 281–301.

—— (1987) Late paraphrenia: phenomenology and etiological factors and their bearing upon problems of the schizophrenic family of disorders. In *Schizophrenia and Aging* (eds N. Miller & G. Cohen), pp. 217–234. New York: Guilford Press.

SHELDRICK, C., JABLENSKY, A. & SARTORIUS, N. (1977) Schizophrenia succeeded by affective illness: catamnestic study and statistical enquiry. *Psychological Medicine*, **7**, 619–624.

SHULMAN, K. & POST, F. (1980) Bipolar affective disorder in old age. *British Journal of Psychiatry*, **136**, 26–32.

TAYLOR, M. A. & ABRAMS, R. (1984) Cognitive impairment in schizophrenia. *American Journal of Psychiatry*, **141**, 196–201.

WADDINGTON, J. L., BROWN, K., O'NEIL, L., *et al* (1989) Cognitive impairment, clinical course and treatment in out-patients with bipolar affective disorder: relationship to tardive dyskinesia. *Psychological Medicine*, **19**, 897–902.

WEINBERGER, D. R. (1987) Implications of normal brain development for the pathogenesis of schizophrenia. *Archives of General Psychiatry*, **44**, 660–669.

WILLIAMS, P. V. & McGLASHAN, T. H. (1987) Schizoaffective psychosis. I. Comparative long-term outcome. *Archives of General Psychiatry*, **44**, 130–137.

WINOKUR, G., SCHARFETTER, C. & ANGST, J. (1985) Stability of psychotic symptomatology (delusions, hallucinations), affective syndromes, and schizophrenic symptoms (thought disorder, incongruent affect) over episodes in remitting psychoses. *European Archives of Psychiatry and Neurological Sciences*, **234**, 303–307.

ZERBIN-RUDIN, E. (1986) Schizoaffective and other atypical psychoses: the genetical aspect. In *Schizoaffective Psychoses* (eds A. Marneros & M. T. Tsuang), pp. 225–231. Berlin: Springer.

9 The affective disorders: bipolar disorder and major depression

MYRNA M. WEISSMAN

The hypothesis examined in this chapter is that bipolar disorder and major depression are discrete rather than continuous disorders. In the absence of understanding of aetiology or pathophysiology, this chapter examines the epidemiology (differential rates and risks) and genetic epidemiology (twin and familial aggregation studies) of bipolar disorder and major depression in the context of two questions. Is there evidence for the separateness of the disorders? Is there utility for these distinctions? I use the American Psychiatric Association's (1980) DSM–III diagnostic criteria rather than its 1987 revision (DSM–III–R), as much of the evidence currently available is based on DSM–III. Moreover, the changes in the revision regarding the affective disorders are relatively minor and will not change the thrust of the discussion. I include research based on Research Diagnostic Criteria (RDC; Spitzer *et al*, 1978) noting Kendell's (1989) comments that RDC, at least in twin studies, were the most sensitive or the most precise constellation in picking out heritability. The evidence presented supports the validity of the separation of bipolar disorder and major depression. The evidence for the validity of the conventional subtypes of major depression based on symptom patterns, such as endogenous subtypes, is not strong. There is uncertainty about which subtype of major depression may be related to bipolar illness.

Historical context

The differentiation of bipolar and unipolar disorder was initially suggested by Kraepelin (1913) in his definition of manic–depressive illness. In Kraepelin's system, monopolar was either recurrent depression or mania, but not both. This concept was elaborated by Leonhard *et al* (1962), who proposed that manic–depression be divided into bipolar and monopolar illness. Bipolar patients were those with a history of both mania and depression, and monopolar included patients with depression only. The

TABLE 9.1
Sample characteristics in five ECA sites in the USA

	New Haven	Baltimore	St Louis	Durham	Los Angeles
Adult population aged 18 + (1980 census)	300 000	175 000	280 000	197 000	246 000
Completed interviews in each site	5034	3481	3004	3921	3132
Completion rate	77%	78%	79%	79%	68%

separation of mania gained acceptance as a useful concept by independent family studies – by Angst (1966) and Perris (1966) – and with the introduction of lithium and its demonstration as an effective treatment for bipolar illness (Keller, 1987; Klerman, 1988). While the term 'bipolar' gained wide acceptance, the concept of unipolar was not adopted in either DSM–III or its revision. The non-bipolar forms were included under the concept of major depression, and subtypes of melancholia and psychotic were added to major depression. There was debate about the validity of the non-bipolar subtypes of major depression and where endogenous and neurotic subtypes belonged. To a great extent, these distinctions and uncertainties still remain.

Epidemiological evidence

Data on the epidemiology of affective disorder using DSM–III based on a probability sample of a community are now available from the Epidemiologic Catchment Area Study (ECA) in the United States. Over 18 000 adults, 18 years of age and over, in five US communities were assessed using Diagnostic Interview Schedule (DIS), which generates DSM–III diagnoses. The full details of design and methods as well as data on the rates of affective disorders have been presented by Regier *et al* (1984) and Weissman *et al* (1988*a*).

Table 9.1 describes the population, sample, and response rates from the five ECA sites. Table 9.2 summarises the rates and characteristics of major depression and bipolar disorder based on the five ECA sites. Weighted rates

TABLE 9.2
Rates and characteristics of subjects with bipolar disorder and major depression in five ECA sites

	Bipolar disorder	Major depression
Lifetime rate per 100 population[1]	1.3	4.7
Six-month rate per 100 population[1]	0.9	2.2
Mean age first onset: years	21.2	27.4
Odds ratio (female : male)	1.2	2.5

1. Weighted.

TABLE 9.3
Summary of concordance rates for bipolar disorder in the twin studies

	Monozygotic	Dizygotic	Investigator
Concordance rate for bipolar disorder	72%	14%	Allen (summary of 10 studies)
	79%	24%	Bertelsen
	75%	0%	Torgersen

Data derived from Torgersen (1986).

are presented since each sample case has a known probability of selection from the target population. A weight is assigned to each respondent to enable compensation for under- or oversampling when determining prevalence. The results clearly show that bipolar disorder and major depression have different prevalence rates, ages of first onset, and sex distribution. The lifetime rates per 100 population of bipolar disorder are 1.3, and, of major depression 4.7. The respective mean ages at first onset are 21 and 27 years. While the sex distribution is equal in bipolar disorder, the rates for major depression are more than twofold higher in women than in men. These different epidemiologies suggest the distinctiveness of these disorders.

Twin studies

As summarised by Torgersen (1986), the twin studies have shown the following.

(a) Heredity contributes to the development of bipolar disorder: there is a higher concordance of bipolar disorder in monozygotic than in dizygotic twins (Table 9.3).

(b) Bipolar disorder and major depression are likely to be separate in that few cotwins of index twins with bipolar disorder have a major depression, and few cotwins of index twins with major depression have a bipolar disorder (Table 9.4). However, more of the monozygotic

TABLE 9.4
Probandwise concordance rates for affective disorders for bipolar disorder and major depression

Proband diagnosis	Cotwin diagnosis		
	bipolar	major depression	other, non-affective disorders
Bipolar disorder			
monozygotic	75%	25%	0%
dizygotic	0%	0%	17%
Major depression			
monozygotic	3%	27%	9%
dizygotic	2%	12%	17%

Data derived from Torgersen (1986).

TABLE 9.5
Probandwise concordance rates for affective disorders by subtype of major depression

Proband diagnosis	Cotwin diagnosis		
	bipolar	major depression	other, non-affective disorders
Psychotic major depressive disorder			
monozygotic	0%	40%	0%
dizygotic	0%	15%	23%
Non-psychotic major depressive disorder			
monozygotic	4%	25%	11%
dizygotic	2%	11%	15%

Data derived from Torgersen (1986).

twins with bipolar disorder have cotwins with major depression than the converse, suggesting partial overlap between these disorders. It is still unclear which subtypes of major depression may be related to bipolar disorder.

(c) The evidence for heritability of major depression is more ambiguous. However, when subtypes of major depression are examined, the best evidence for heritability is for psychotic major depression, where concordance rates in monozygotic twins are higher than for non-psychotic major depression (Table 9.5). (This finding is consistent with the family data of Leckman *et al* (1984).)

(d) There is little evidence for the heritability of other, non-affective psychiatric disorders in cotwins of probands with bipolar disorder, major depression, psychotic, or non-psychotic depressive types (Table 9.5).

It should be emphasised, however, that the number of twin studies using RDC or DSM–III criteria are small and that more work in this area is needed.

Family studies

Family studies are useful for studying the overlap and independence of disorders. Independence is assessed by studying the cross-prevalence of one illness in relatives of probands with the second illness. If the two illnesses are independent, the cross-prevalences are the same as in the controls or the population prevalence. If they are not independent, either or both of the cross-prevalences may be higher.

The findings for family studies partially parallel those of the twin studies, as follows (see the Weissman-Gershon family study (Table 9.6) for illustration and Weissman *et al* (1984) for details of methods).

TABLE 9.6

Lifetime rates per 100 population[1] of psychiatric disorders in first-degree relatives of probands with bipolar disorder, major depression or normal controls in two studies

	Proband group			
	Gershon et al *(1987)*		Weissman et al *(1988*a,b*)*	
Relatives' diagnosis	*bipolar disorder*	*major depressive disorder*	*major depressive disorder[2]*	*normal controls*
Schizophrenia	0.2	0.0	0.4	0.2
Bipolar I disorder	4.9	1.5	0.8	0.2
Major depressive disorder	14.3	16.8	18.4	5.9
Cyclothymia	3.0	0.0	0.7	0.0
Hyperthymia	2.8	1.8	0.4	0.6
Anxiety disorder	1.2	2.4	6.9	2.9
Substance abuse	4.9	7.3	6.3	5.8
Any psychiatric disorder	50.1	52.7	50.2	25.8

1.   Age-adjusted rate with diagnostic hierarchies.
2.   Only probands admitted to hospital are included so that groups are comparable between studies.

(a) The rates of bipolar disorder are consistently higher in relatives of affectively ill probands than in relatives of controls.

(b) There are increased rates of major depression in the relatives of probands with bipolar disorder, although the reverse is generally not found. This implies a partial overlap between bipolar disorder and major depression.

(c) As in the epidemiological studies, the rates of bipolar disorder in relatives were equal in males and females and the rates of major depression were higher in females.

(d) Schizophrenia, alcohol abuse, and a host of other disorders did *not* show familial aggregation with affective disorders. This has also been found by others (Merikangas *et al*, 1985). Although bipolar disorder and alcoholism commonly occur in the same individual, alcoholism by itself does not appear to co-segregate in the relatives of probands with bipolar disorder or major depression, suggesting that alcoholism does not appear to belong in the genetic spectrum of bipolar disorder (Angst, 1966, 1973).

(e) The findings for cyclothymia, hyperthymia, and dysthymia are quite different and suggest that they may be on the spectrum of bipolar disorder and major depression. They may be mild manifestations or the sequelae of major depression or bipolar disorder. Some support for this idea comes from clinical follow-up studies, which indicate that many patients with major depression or bipolar disorder go on to develop these milder forms of illness (Akiskal *et al*, 1981).

(f) There is not an increase in overall rates of psychiatric disorder in the relatives of the probands with bipolar as compared with major depression, suggesting that bipolar disorder does *not* represent a division on a continuum of severity. The overall risk of psychiatric illness is comparable in the relatives of probands with bipolar disorder and major depression. The hypothesis for gradients or a continuum of liability going from severe bipolar disorder to a more mild form of affective disorder or major depression is not supported.

(g) Schizophrenia is not increased in the relatives of probands with affective disorders as compared with relatives of normal controls. Studies that show an increased risk of affective disorders in relatives of probands with schizophrenia may do so because of the absence of control groups. Affective disorders have a relatively high population prevalence, so one would expect to find a substantial rate of affective disorders by chance only. Control groups can answer questions about the rates of increase, over and above what might be expected by chance.

The relationship between major depression and bipolar disorder

While there is evidence for the separation of bipolar disorder from major depression – as proposed by Leonhard, Angst, and others, and in DSM–III as noted above – the data from these studies are ambiguous. Major depression is increased in the first-degree relatives of probands with bipolar disorder or major depression, but the converse is not true. There is considerably less evidence and consensus on the heterogeneity of major depression and on what subtype of major depression may be related to bipolar disorder. This is an area requiring further research. It is interesting to note that in the family studies, the methods proposed by Kendell (1989) to test the validity of subtypes have been used. That is, a variety of operational criteria, narrow in sequence, with and without comorbidity, have been used in both the proband groups and their relatives to determine "with some precision which syndromes co-aggregate and how broadly it is possible to define individual categories . . . without their propensity to breed true breaking down".

Evidence that specific subtypes increase rates of a particular disorder suggests the validity or utility of the subtypes. If a particular subtype increases the risk of another disorder, this suggests its relationship to that disorder. The family studies suggest that the evidence for the current conventional subtypes based on symptom patterns are not as strong as the evidence for the validity of separation of bipolar disorder and major depression.

Testing the validity of subtypes

Table 9.7 illustrates our efforts to test the validity of subtypes of major depression and to determine the relationship, if any, between particular subtypes of major depression and bipolar disorder. The data were derived from a family study of 1331 first-degree relatives of 215 probands with major depression or normal controls (Weissman *et al*, 1984, 1988*b*; Leckman *et al*, 984). The lack of an increase in the risk of major depression in relatives

TABLE 9.7

Lifetime rates per 100 population and odds ratio[1] of major depression and bipolar disorder by subtype of major depression in proband

| | Diagnosis in relatives | | | |
| | Major depression | | Bipolar disorder | |
Subtype of major depression in proband	lifetime rates	odds ratio	lifetime rates	odds ratio
RDC endogenous	16.3	1.2	0.7	0.9
DSM–III melancholia	17.5	1.2	1.1	2.4
RDC delusional	19.6	1.5	2.3*	6.5

1. Odds ratio compares rate of disorder in relatives of proband with and without specific subtype controlling for age, sex and interview status of relative.
* $P < 0.05$.

of probands with endogenous or melancholic depression, as shown in Table 9.7, has also been shown in family studies reported by Andreasen *et al* (1986), Zimmerman *et al* (1986), and in the original studies by Angst (1966, 1973). While there was little evidence that the subtypes increased the risk of major depression overall, the occurrence of a delusional subtype in probands increased the risk of bipolar disorder in adult relatives. These latter findings were replicated in a sample of 220 children (6–23 years of age) from this study (Weissman *et al*, 1988*b*). There was also evidence for the specificity of delusional depression in relatives. The suggestion that delusional depression may be a specific subtype and may be related to bipolar disorders requires follow-up – particularly in light of Torgersen's (1986) twin study, which suggests that delusional depression was a more heritable form of major depression.

Conclusion and alternative explanations for the continuum hypothesis

Data from epidemiological, family, and twin studies support the utility of separation of bipolar disorder and major depression and some overlap between them. Both major depression and bipolar disorder are probably heterogeneous, and there is evidence for a relationship between delusional subtypes of major depression and bipolar disorder (Weissman *et al* (1988*b*) review other evidence).

Some of the evidence for the continuum hypothesis of major psychoses could have alternative explanations. For example, the increased rates of illness by generation have been proposed by Crow (1986) as evidence of changing mutations. However, this phenomenon could be explained by the cohort effect – the increasing rates of major depression and bipolar disorders in the cohort born since World War II – which has been noted now in several family and epidemiological studies in many, but not all, countries reporting data (Klerman *et al*, 1985; Gershon *et al*, 1987; Klerman & Weissman, 1989; Lasch *et al*, 1990). A cohort effect could be explained by historical and environmental changes as well as changing mutations.

The evidence that major depression can be found in the families of schizophrenics could be explained by the absence of control groups in family studies reporting high rates of depression and also by assortative mating. Major depression is a high-prevalence disorder; therefore, elevated rates in the families of probands with any psychiatric disorder are to be expected. Control groups are necessary in order to determine whether the observed increase in the families of ill probands is over and above what might be expected by chance. Moreover, there is evidence that psychiatric patients assortatively cross-mate. If a schizophrenic and depressed proband mate, one would expect to find increased rates of both disorders in the offspring.

In summary, the elegant genetic models proposed by Dr Crow (Chapter 3) and others may well turn out to be the correct ones. With more sophisticated technologies becoming available for studying the aetiology of the major psychoses, particularly the molecular genetic methods, all of our concepts of the mental disorders and their relationship to one another may be revised. Currently, however, genetic linkage studies of psychiatric disorders require precise defining of the phenotype in ways which may suggest aetiological homogeneity. In the absence of sufficient evidence to the contrary, the division of bipolar and non-bipolar major depression and the search for subtypes of major depression, which are on the spectrum of bipolar disorders, may provide more precision. However, no reasonable hypothesis about a diagnostic classification should be precluded from testing, provided that the hypothesis about a diagnostic classification is specified *a priori* and diagnoses are applied without knowledge of the biological outcome.

References

AKISKAL, H. S., BITAR, A. H., PUZANTIAN, V. R., *et al* (1981) Subaffective disorders: dysthymic, cyclothymic, and bipolar II disorders in the "borderline" realm. *Psychiatric Clinics of North America*, **4**, 25–46.

AMERICAN PSYCHIATRIC ASSOCIATION (1980) *Diagnostic and Statistical Manual of Mental Disorders* (3rd edn) (DSM–III). Washington, DC: APA.

ANDREASEN, N. C., SCHEFTNER, W., REICH, T., *et al* (1986) The validation of the concept of endogenous depression: a family study approach. *Archives of General Psychiatry*, **43**, 246–251.

ANGST, J. (1966) *Zur Ätiologie und Nosologie endogener depressiver Psychosen*. Berlin-Heidelberg: Springer-Verlag.

—— (1973) The etiology and nosology of endogenous depressive psychoses. *Foreign Psychiatry*, **2**, 1–108.

CROW, T. J. (1986) The continuum of psychosis and its implication for the structure of the gene. *British Journal of Psychiatry*, **149**, 419–429.

GERSHON, E., HAMOVIT, J., GURROFF, J., et al (1987) Birth-cohort changes in manic and depressive disorders in relatives of bipolar and schizoaffective patients. *Archives of General Psychiatry*, **44**, 314–319.

KENDELL, R. E. (1989) Clinical validity. *Psychological Medicine*, **19**, 45–55.

KLERMAN, G. L., LAVORI, P. W., RICE, J., et al (1985) Birth cohort trends in rates of major depressive disorder among relatives of patients with affective disorder. *Archives of General Psychiatry*, **42**, 689–693.

——— & WEISSMAN, M. M. (1989) Increasing rates of depression. *Journal of the American Medical Association*, **261**, 229–235.

KRAEPELIN, E. (1913) Das manisch–depressive Irresein. In *Psychiatrie: Ein Lehrbuch für Studierende und Ärzte* (8th edn), vol. III, part 2, pp. 1183–1395. Leipzig: Barth.

LASCH, K., WEISSMAN, M. M., WICKRAMARATNE, P. J., et al (1990) Birth cohort changes in the rates of mania. *Psychiatry Research*, **33**, 31–37.

LECKMAN, J. F., WEISSMAN, M. M., PRUSOFF, B. A., et al (1984) Subtypes of depression. Family study perspective. *Archives of General Psychiatry*, **41**, 833–838.

LEONHARD, K., KORFF, I. & SCHULTZ, H. (1962) Die Temperamente in den Familien der monopolaren und bipolaren phasischen Psychosen. *Psychiatric Neurology*, **143**, 416–434.

MERIKANGAS, K. R., LECKMAN, M. D., PRUSOFF, B. A., et al (1985) Familial transmission of depression and alcoholism. *Archives of General Psychiatry*, **42**, 367–372.

PERRIS, C. (1966) A study of bipolar (manic depressive) and unipolar recurrent depressive psychoses. *Acta Psychiatrica Scandinavica*, **194**, 1–194.

REGIER, D. A., MYERS, J. K., KRAMER, M., et al (1984) The NIMH Epidemiologic Catchment Area program: historical context, major objectives, and study population characteristics. *Archives of General Psychiatry*, **41**, 934–941.

SPITZER, R. L., ENDICOTT, J. & ROBINS, E. (1978) *Research Diagnostic Criteria for a Selected Group of Functional Disorders* (3rd edn). New York: New York State Psychiatric Institute.

TORGERSEN, S. (1986) Genetic factors in moderately severe and mild affective disorders. *Archives of General Psychiatry*, **43**, 222–226.

WEISSMAN, M. M., GERSHON, E. S., KIDD, K. K., et al (1984) Psychiatric disorders in the relatives of probands with affective disorders. The Yale University–National Institute of Mental Health Collaborative Study. *Archives of General Psychiatry*, **41**, 13–21.

———, LEAF, P. L., TISCHLER, G. L., et al (1988a) Affective disorders in five United States communities. *Psychological Medicine*, **18**, 141–153.

———, WARNER, V., JOHN, K., et al (1988b) Delusional depression and bipolar spectrum: evidence for a possible association from a family study of children. *Neuropsychopharmacology*, **1**, 257–264.

ZIMMERMAN, M., CORYELL, W., PFOHL, B., et al (1986) The validity of four definitions of endogenous depression. II. Clinical, demographic, familial, and psychosocial correlates. *Archives of General Psychiatry*, **43**, 234–244.

10 Neuroses and personality disorders

PETER TYRER

The general feature of modern classification in psychiatry to become more agnostic and atheoretical is well illustrated in the descriptions of the neuroses and personality disorders. As a reaction to the unsatisfactory aetiological hypotheses of psychoanalysis, the word 'neurosis' has been ejected altogether from the new classifications. However, the expulsion of one naughty boy from the school does not mean that deviance has been eliminated, and the concept of neurosis still remains in the background to haunt its detractors (Bayer & Spitzer, 1985). By contrast, personality disorders have come into their own in the past few years since the introduction of DSM–III (American Psychiatric Association, 1980) gave them new respect and emphasised the importance of personality status as a separate axis of classification.

The introduction of operational criteria into the classification of disorders, which were previously served only by diffuse description, has also been a major boost to their respectability. This is illustrated by the number of publications that are now appearing on personality disorder in its own right. Before 1980 personality disorders were discussed in most psychiatric texts together with the neuroses (as indeed they are in this chapter) because, although personality disorders did not appear to belong anywhere, they seem to show greater parallels with the neuroses through their frequent descriptions in the psychodynamic literature. Now it is appreciated that personality disorder belongs no more with neuroses than it does with disorders such as schizophrenia; these disorders need to be discussed in their own right, independently of mental state ones.

Before 1980 and the introduction of DSM–III, the diagnoses encapsulating the neuroses were, broadly:

(a) agoraphobia
(b) social phobia
(c) simple phobia
(d) obsessive–compulsive disorder
(e) depressive neurosis.

In contrast, the new diagnoses basically comprise:

(a) generalised anxiety disorder
(b) panic disorder
(c) dysthymic disorder
(d) somatoform disorder
(e) depressive episode.

These are elaborated upon, along with stress-related disorders and personality disorders, in Table 10.1. Many readers in Britain will find some of the new nomenclature strange. Panic disorder is a recent introduction from the USA and still greeted with scepticism in some quarters; somatoform disorder, quite apart from being a polysyllabic mouthful, is virtually unknown to the average European clinician, and some of the personality disorders (e.g. anxious (avoidant), schizotypal) will appear equally strange.

The advantages and disadvantages of these newer concepts are discussed in this chapter.

The absence of theory

One of the major handicaps of the theoretical superstructure of neuroses has been its unreliability. Unfortunately the arguments used by psychoanalysts in explaining symptoms are unsatisfactory as scientific concepts. It will quickly be apparent to anyone versed in scientific method that a theoretical system which allows one set of symptoms or beliefs to indicate a specific diagnosis while allowing the opposite set of symptoms and beliefs to indicate the same diagnosis (by reaction formation) is more than unsatisfactory – it is a travesty of knowledge. The mental mechanisms used to explain symptom formation and psychodynamic theory are so flexible that all hypotheses can be proved. Thus, like the dodo in Carroll's *Through the Looking Glass*, all theories have won and "all shall have prizes". The psychodynamicist may argue that these mechanisms are true in clinical practice by recalling case histories; however, these are really no more than anecdotes and do not give them any status as explanatory scientific concepts.

When using operational criteria to define the neurotic disorders the diagnostician is left in no doubt about whether or not the requirements for a particular category are satisfied. This is helped even more by concentrating on the presenting symptoms in reaching decisions about classification. These are expressed directly by the patient and require no special interpretation. Indeed, lay interviewers can be trained to administer interview schedules that categorise symptoms according to the appropriate diagnoses. The Diagnostic Interview Schedule (DIS; Robins *et al*, 1979) is perhaps the best known of these.

TABLE 10.1
Comparison of current classification of personality disorder

ICD–10		DSM–III–R	
Description	*Code*	*Description*	*Code*
Paranoid – excessive sensitivity, suspiciousness, preoccupation with conspiratorial explanation of events, with a persistent tendency to self-reference	F60.0	Paranoid – interpretation of people's actions as deliberately demeaning or threatening	301.00
Schizoid – emotional coldness, detachment, lack of interest in other people, eccentricity and introspective fantasy	F60.1	Schizoid – indifference to relationships and restricted range of emotional experience and expression	301.20
No equivalent		Schizotypal – deficit in inter-personal relatedness with peculiarities of ideation, appearance and behaviour	302.22
Anankastic – indecisiveness, doubt, excessive caution, pedantry, rigidity and need to plan in immaculate detail	F60.5	Obsessive–compulsive – pervasive perfectionism and inflexibility	301.40
Histrionic – self-dramatisation, shallow mood, egocentricity and craving for excitement with persistent manipulative behaviour	F60.4	Histrionic – excessive emotionally and attention-seeking	301.50
Dependent – failure to take responsibility for actions, with subordination of personal needs to those of others, excessive dependence with need for constant reassurance and feelings of helplessness when a close relationship ends	F60.7	Dependent – persistent dependent and submissive behaviour	301.60
Dyssocial – callous unconcern for others, with irresponsibility, irritability and aggression, and incapacity to maintain enduring relationships	F60.2	Antisocial – evidence of repeated conduct disorder before the age of 15 years	301.70
No equivalent		Narcissistic – pervasive grandiosity, lack of empathy, and hypersensitivity to the evaluation of others	301.81
Anxious – persistent tension, self-consciousness, exaggeration of risks and dangers, hyper-sensitivity to rejection, and restricted lifestyle because of insecurity	F60.6	Avoidant – pervasive social discomfort, fear of negative evaluation and timidity	301.82
Impulsive – inability to control anger, to plan ahead, or to think before acts, with unpredictable mood and quarrelsome behaviour	F60.30[1]	Borderline – pervasive instability of mood, and self-image	301.83

continued

ICD-10		DSM-III-R	
Description	Code	Description	Code
Borderline – unclear self-image, involvement in intense and unstable relationships	F60.31[1]	Passive – aggressive/pervasive passive resistance to demands for adequate social and occupational performance	301.84

1. Included under heading of emotionally labile personality disorder.

The same principle applies to the classification of personality disorders. Although the categorisation of behaviour is a little more difficult than that of symptoms, the operational criteria for personality disorders concentrate on well defined examples of abnormal elements of behaviour. These "prototypic acts" (Blashfield *et al*, 1985) can almost be regarded as pathognomonic of the disorder being studied and are worthy of accurate delineation because they represent pure examples of the disorder under scrutiny.

By using operational criteria the decision about categorisation is made easily, without the vagaries of clinical judgement, as once a subject has satisfied the necessary minimum of criteria the diagnosis is applied automatically. Thus a population is obtained which is homogeneous with regard to the operational criteria, and if they have been chosen correctly, this should represent a single disorder. Once this has been done disorders can be compared, for example with regard to the amount of social dysfunction each of them produces. This has been particularly valuable in the US, where each disorder has had a financial tag attached to it so that the handicap it produces can be quantitatively assessed for insurance purposes.

Using these new systems nothing is hidden. The classification depends on what is exhibited in terms of behaviour and symptoms and there is no necessity for discussions about 'unconscious' motivation and other inaccessible information which was formerly so important in making the diagnoses, and which made psychiatrists so prone to destruction by cross-examination in courts of law.

Although this absence of theory may be an unqualified bonus to the nosologist it falls down with some disorders, notably those that used to be classified together under the rubric of 'hysteria'. These have now been split up (appropriately enough, as hysteria is characteristically a splitting disorder) between the somatoform and dissociative disorders, and no longer have any common features. This is perhaps predictable, as Freud and his followers erected the superstructure of psychoanalysis on the somewhat shaky base of hysteria and generalised from this to all neurotic disorders, so that this condition has suffered most under the new classification regime. However, if one accepts the concept of hysteria as a condition that simulates other psychiatric and physical disorders, a classification that is based entirely on symptoms will fail to separate hysterical symptoms from those that are not simulated (consciously or unconsciously). The new classification is uncomfortable over this issue but makes some allowance for the problem by bringing in the concept of 'psychosocial stressors' when discussing dissociative and somatoform disorders. However, this is quite different from seeing the manifestation of the symptoms as an understandable event in a "life story" (Slavney, 1990), in which a large amount of information available from a detailed psychiatric history can help to explain the onset of what otherwise would be regarded as symptoms of a quite different disorder.

The atheoretical stance also does not apply to the stress and adjustment disorders. Here it is assumed, probably correctly, that the symptoms would not have arisen but for the experience of a major life event or a similar set of circumstances. The nature of the stressor determines whether the condition is classified as an acute stress (appearing only in the World Health Organization's (1988) ICD-10), adjustment or post-traumatic stress disorder. While it may be argued that the attribution of a causal link between these particular stressors and symptoms does not involve theory, this can be disputed and in any case leads to difficulties in classification. Thus, for example, panic is regarded as a major symptom of both adjustment and post-traumatic stress disorder. The qualifying criteria for a separate diagnosis of panic disorder are relatively low, as, for example in DSM-III-R (American Psychiatric Association, 1987), the appearance of a single panic attack followed by a continual fear of having another is sufficient to satisfy the diagnosis. The clinician is not helped to make the distinction between panic disorder in the setting of an adjustment disorder and that which occurs independently. In both instances the panic almost invariably comes on without an obvious external cue and the symptoms are identical.

The overlap between categories

It is recognised that identification of a homogeneous population for one or more groups of clinical symptoms does not prevent overlap with others. Nevertheless, the identification of groups that are homogeneous with respect to at least one group of characteristics is the first step in effecting separation from others.

In practical terms the overlap is not as significant as it first appears. Thus, for example, the frequent association of anxiety and depression is not a problem to many clinicians. Depression leads to greater social dysfunction than anxiety (e.g. Casey *et al*, 1985), and so it is more reasonable to concentrate on treating the depressive symptoms and to regard the anxiety as only of secondary importance.

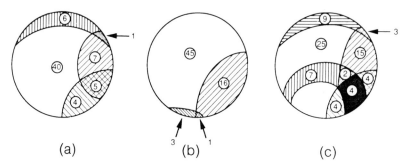

Fig. 10.1. *Overlap of diagnoses in 201 patients according to the Structured Interview Schedule for DSM–III (SCID): (a) 63 with dysthymia, (b) 65 with generalised anxiety disorder, and (c) 73 with panic disorder (□ generalised anxiety, ▨ simple phobia, ▧ social phobia, ▤ panic, ▥ dysthymia)*

The imposition of what is, in effect, a hierarchy of symptoms is even more apparent when a condition such as obsessive–compulsive disorder is being considered. Thus, for example, the obsessive–compulsive patient who carries out repeated washing rituals because of fear of a terrible disaster if these are not performed is treated for the ritualistic behaviour rather than the accompanying anxiety. One of the common treatments given – response prevention – obviously takes into account the anxiety, but it would be quite inappropriate for the anxiety to be considered as the primary phenomenon.

The disadvantages of overlap are immediately obvious. Firstly, the identification of homogeneous groups is undermined, as illustrated by the Venn diagrams in Fig. 10.1, which show the degree of overlap between DSM–III diagnoses for neurotic disorder (Tyrer *et al*, 1988). The problem is made more serious if cross-sectional overlap (comparison at one point in time) is accompanied by temporal instability (changing of symptoms and overlap over time). Thus if a patient showing all the characteristics for homogeneous diagnosis A presents six months later with all the characteristics sufficient for the diagnosis of homogeneous diagnosis B, the separation of A and B may be threatened. However, if the change from A to B is consistent, this can be acknowledged by combined diagnoses such as with manic–depressive psychosis or bipolar affective disorders.

With the neuroses, however, the difficulties in classification are compounded by the persistent co-occurrence of the main disorders (anxiety, depression, phobias, somatoform and dissociative disorders) (Boyd *et al*, 1984). If one disorder progressed predictably to another, such as the path postulated by Klein (1981) for panic disorder developing to agoraphobia with panic, the alteration in diagnosis would not be inconsistent. Detailed follow-up studies, however, have shown that the diagnoses change frequently and show no pattern that could in any way be interpreted as progression of disorder (Tyrer *et al*, 1987). In a project in which continuous assessment of symptoms and service use is being made over five years, we compared the psychopathology and diagnostic change in patients diagnosed as having dysthymia, generalised anxiety disorder and panic disorder using DSM–III criteria formalised in a structured interview schedule (Spitzer & Williams, 1983). Very little clinical difference was shown between the three diagnostic groups over time, apart from the finding that panic had quantitatively more severe anxiety than generalised anxiety disorder (Tyrer *et al*, 1988, 1990). Diagnostic change was frequent, with only 19% of patients with generalised anxiety disorder, 14% of those with dysthymia and 5% of those with panic disorder retaining their original diagnosis (or improving to no diagnosis) in the first two years of follow-up (Seivewright & Tyrer, 1990).

The pattern shown by personality disorders also shows many similarities with those of the neuroses. There is a tremendous degree of overlap between different types of personality disorder (which is entirely predictable in view of the overlap between the operational criteria) (Livesley & Jackson, 1986), and as no hierarchy is adopted in classifying personality disorder in DSM–III and DSM–III–R (apart from relegating passive aggressive personality disorder to a lower position in DSM–III) there is no structure that allows comparison between the different categories. It is reasonable to suppose that a patient who satisfies the criteria for six personality disorders is more disturbed than one who just satisfies the criteria for one, but this is ignored as the whole purpose of this classification is to provide a useful qualitative categorisation once the diagnostic boundary of personality disorder has been reached.

Borderline personality disorder is the most notorious in this respect; indeed it is difficult to study any population of personality disorders in the US without finding that borderline diagnoses are prominent. When the co-occurrence of borderline and histrionic personality disorders is as high as 46% (Widiger & Rodgers, 1989) it is reasonable to question the value of keeping the diagnoses separate.

Although mental state diagnoses are kept separate from personality disorders in the new classifications, it is important to recognise that the simultaneous presence of a personality and a neurotic disorder is common. The typical patient with a neurotic disorder is much more likely to have what used to be called an 'oral' personality (which more recently is classified among the dependent or anankastic categories) than other personality disorders (Lazare *et al*, 1976; Tyrer *et al*, 1983, 1986). A similar association has been noted between depressive disorders and borderline personality disorder (Pope *et al*, 1983; McGlashan, 1983).

When these associations are sufficiently frequent as to be the norm, it is reasonable to consider combining the diagnoses of personality disorder and mental state. This should not be confined to neurotic disorders. Although there is merit in separating mental state from the personality domain, this should not blind us to the advantages of combining diagnoses when associations are strong. Two associations that deserve further inquiry are a combination of neurotic disorders with dependent personality and that between borderline personality disorder and depression. The first has been described as the "general neurotic syndrome" (Tyrer, 1985) and the concept has been supported by several studies, including epidemiological (Uhlenhuth *et al*, 1983), clinical (Tyrer *et al*, 1987, 1988) and genetic (Andrews *et al*, 1990). The general neurotic syndrome is argued to be a condition that manifests different neurotic symptoms at different times and pursues a relapsing course, often dependent on the nature of life events experienced, but which generally has a poor prognosis. The alternative, milder, mixed anxiety/depressive disorder, termed 'cothymia' (Tyrer, 1989), carries a better prognosis.

To many who have striven so hard to separate neurotic disorders in the past decade this suggestion appears to be sacrilege. However, in arguing for the acceptance of such a syndrome, I would ask that the classification system at least allows such combination of symptoms (and personality characteristics) to be classified. At present the classification allows no such combination of personality and mental symptoms, and is extraordinarily reluctant to allow mixed anxiety/depressive disorders. The barest chink of acceptance has been shown in the recent draft ICD–10 classification, which allows mixed anxiety/depressive disorder a separate classification. However, this particular diagnosis is so minor that it barely deserves to be classified at all, because if patients qualify for a separate anxiety or depressive disorder separately this should take precedence (World Health Organization, 1988).

The combination of borderline personality disorder and depression is sufficiently common to suggest that a 'borderline syndrome' should be described rather than a specific personality disorder (Tyrer, 1989). The merit of combining the depressed mood with the personality disturbance is that the depression in borderline personality appears to be quite different from depression in other conditions. It is often brief and intense, associated with impulsive suicide attempts, and responds at least as well to low doses of antipsychotic medication as it does to conventional antidepressant therapy (Soloff *et al*, 1986). Again, I am not arguing for uncritical acceptance of a new 'syndrome' (a category under the heading of 'personality diathesis' may be necessary to indicate a combined personality/mental-state diagnosis in which the presence of a personality disorder makes the patient vulnerable to a named mental illness), but to state the case for an appropriate structure of classification that allows such combined conditions to be classified in future. At present there is no room for these combined conditions and it is fair to ask whether this rigidity by psychiatric nosologists might be because of fear that such combined syndromes might be diagnosed so much more frequently than the 'pure' states in current use that the latter might disappear altogether.

The separate classification of depression

In both ICD-10 and DSM-III-R depression is categorised in a separate section on mood disorders. The advantages of this revision of classification (which is a major change from previous ones) is that the clinician who wants to classify a depressive disorder knows exactly where to look. In earlier classifications depression could be classified in almost any part of the classification system and this made no sense. It is perhaps significant that in the "Mental Health Enquiry" (Department of Health and Social Security, 1989), the national register for the recording of psychiatric diagnoses of patients who have been admitted to hospital, a consistent majority of patients with depression (around 55%) are included under the heading of "not otherwise classified". This suggests that the diagnostic system was causing confusion and it was very difficult to interpret the labels given by psychiatrists in classifying patients into the important major diagnoses.

One other reason for classifying all depressive disorders together is that the major distinction made between categories such as 'endogenous' and 'reactive' had been shown to be flawed in most of the research inquiries carried out into the validity of this separation (e.g. Kendell, 1976). The new classifications merely make a distinction between mild, moderate and severe depressions and between single and recurrent episodes, and carry an additional grouping indicating the presence or absence of both somatic and psychotic symptoms. Thus the concept of depressive 'neurosis' belonging with the neurotic disorders has been removed from the new classification. This type of depression now has to be given a different name (it is misleadingly called 'dysthymia' in the American system) because the words 'depressive' and 'neurosis' together constitute an oxymoron in modern psychiatric parlance, a combination of words that is contradictory.

Any classification based on clinical practice recognises this distinction as nonsensical. While recognising the advantages of keeping all depressive disorders together, the extensive overlap between anxiety and depression, already referred to, means that the dividing line between 'mood' (depressive) and 'non-mood' (anxiety and other emotions) disorders becomes an arbitrary one. It is also ridiculous to remove the concept of depression from the separate group of 'neurotic and stress-related disorders'. Depression is one of the most common symptoms after stress, and to remove it from the classification as soon as it becomes a significant or persistent symptom is extremely difficult to sustain. A unitary concept such as the general neurotic syndrome defines a group of people who are susceptible to neurotic symptoms because of the structure of their personality and related factors, and who demonstrate different symptoms at different times because of the nature of the life events they experience. It is well established that depression is a symptom following loss and that anxiety is one associated with threat and danger, and the study of life events confirms this link (Finlay-Jones & Brown, 1981). Thus the patient with a neurotic diathesis would be likely to have a pathological anxiety reaction when put under any degree of threat and danger (certainly at a level much lower than would justify the label of 'stress disorder', or 'adjustment disorder') and similarly would experience pathological depression when faced with relatively minor loss. What is the advantage of classifying the former among the neuroses and stress-related disorders and to reclassify the patient completely when the danger is replaced by loss and depression as a consequence? When faced with the consequences of bringing all the depressive disorders together in one group the system's handicaps are major, and it is difficult to see it persisting.

Treatment

Even if all the other criticisms of the new classifications were substantiated, if it predicted the outcome of treatment or in other ways was useful as a prognostic indicator, then the classification could still be justified. This is because treatment is by far the most important corollary of diagnosis for the working clinician. I once worked for a clinician who made his diagnoses in retrospect from the effects of treatment. The classification was a simple one and easily summarised as ''treatment-x responsive condition'', where x was the therapeutic agent. While this approach cannot be recommended in its entirety (not least because it would mean that reclassification would depend entirely on changes in treatment), it does have an undeniable attraction.

One of the major reasons behind the new classification of neurotic disorders (and indeed of personality disorders) has been the implication that there is a specific treatment for the diagnosis in question that justifies the use of the diagnostic label. This is all consistent with the atheoretical approach. If this approach is successful in identifying homogeneous syndromes, then it is to be expected that they are different in several major respects and should therefore respond differently to treatment. The atheoretical approach gives no indication which treatment is indicated for which condition but empirical studies can establish this independently.

It is worthwhile looking at each of the major treatments available for neurotic disorder to see whether classification has been of value in selecting appropriate treatment. In evaluating the evidence we are faced immediately by the lack of adequate comparisons across diagnoses. Early trials were carried out with patients across broad diagnostic groupings, and these were followed by similar studies comparing treatments of better-defined diagnoses. However, the obvious need to compare treatments between as well as within specific diagnostic groups has been neglected for reasons that are commercial rather than scientific.

Psychotherapy

Psychotherapists, particularly those who practise the more analytical varieties, have always been sceptical about the value of symptoms in making diagnoses. Symptom presentation is regarded as superficial, though may provide clues to underlying conflict and causation; in themselves they are not considered to be much value. Added to this is a long-standing belief, never satisfactorily confirmed in research studies, that if symptom relief is provided without attention to the underlying conflict then symptoms will re-emerge in another form – the well known theory of symptom substitution.

The psychotherapist therefore predicts that if specific treatments are given for specific neurotic diagnoses there will be a round of diagnostic change in treatment rather like a Scottish dance, in which each diagnostic and treatment couple rotate round the floor, exchanging partners before arriving back in the same place.

Psychotherapists are therefore unwilling to attribute any significance to specific symptoms when it comes to treatment. They pay much greater attention to the phenomenon of personality disorder and, indeed, much of the interest in the subject in the past 20 years has been stimulated by psychotherapists elaborating and defining interesting new concepts. These have mainly been concerned with borderline and Narcissistic personality disorders (Kohut, 1971; Kernberg, 1975). These formulate a structure of personality and give a working model for the psychotherapist in tackling the otherwise inchoate and confusing levels at which patients seem to engage in therapy. However, other types of personality disorder have attracted much less interest from psychotherapists.

Drug treatment

There is a great deal of interest in the drug treatment of neurotic disorder and whether refinement of diagnosis can lead to better selection from the many drugs available. Early attempts to identify treatment-response groups by biochemical tests, including the measurement of amine metabolites in urine, the dexamethasone suppression test and platelet monoamine oxidase levels, have all proved unsatisfactory in predicting response to treatment. Physiological measures such as the electroencephalogram and forearm blood flow have also had their advocates but have not been of particular value in selecting treatment.

The new atheoretical approach to diagnosis in which symptoms dominate the diagnostic picture has been regarded with excitement by the pharmaceutical industry, because if specific diagnoses are related to particular drug treatments this would be of major commercial value. In the 1950s and '60s the main treatments available for the neuroses were: amphetamines and their congeners, which appeared to be effective against neurotic anxiety and depression but could not be continued for any length of time because of addiction; the benzodiazepines, which appeared to be effective in anxiety only; and antidepressants, which were specific for depressive symptoms. The early studies also appeared to suggest that monoamine oxidase inhibitors, the original antidepressants, were not effective in treating severe depression (Medical Research Council, 1965) and should be replaced in favour of tricyclic antidepressants.

These suggestions were made without adequate study of the population that could be loosely included under the title 'neuroses'. Almost all studies were with hospital in-patients or the more severely ill, and although these showed apparently important differences when similar studies were carried out in general practice, there were surprisingly few differences between the different treatments available. At the time it seemed reasonable to ascribe these different findings to differences in methods and unsatisfactory diagnostic practice.

The major breakthrough was made in 1964 by Donald Klein when he suggested that an antidepressant, imipramine, was effective in treating anxiety associated with agoraphobia (Klein, 1964). He subsequently elaborated the view that imipramine acted by blocking acute attacks of anxiety, or panics, and left generalised anxiety unaffected (Klein, 1981). Imipramine therefore seemed to have the property of separating one type of anxiety from another, treating it specifically. This phenomenon, termed "pharmacological dissection" by Klein, became a potent tool in investigating both new drugs and new diagnoses.

The view therefore developed that there was a clear-cut relationship between diagnosis and treatment; that depression should be treated with antidepressants, generalised anxiety with benzodiazepines or other sedatives, and panic anxiety with antidepressants also. All the earlier studies were done with imipramine and Klein's group has continued to work mainly with this compound, but similar findings have been found with other tricyclic antidepressants (Liebowitz *et al*, 1988) and more recently with newer selective serotonin reuptake inhibitors such as fluvoxamine (Montgomery, 1990). If anxiety developed to agoraphobia and persistent avoidance became established, it was appropriate to treat the patient primarily with behaviour therapy such as desensitisation or gradual exposure. However, if panic attacks and agoraphobia were present together, antidepressants alone would treat all the symptoms, since the phobia could be seen as secondary to the panic, with avoidance simply a manoeuvre to reduce the vulnerability of the patient during a panic attack (Klein, 1981).

Unfortunately all these predictions were made without the studies that are necessary to establish the validity of these hypotheses. If it is argued that response to treatment is dependent on diagnosis, it behoves the investigator to test the treatment in a range of diagnoses simultaneously. Thus diagnosis can be examined as a predictor of response. Despite the merits of this approach there have been very few studies using this design in which different diagnoses as well as different treatments are compared. However, all of those that have been carried out have thrown doubt both on the diagnostic separation of neurotic depression and anxiety, and between panic and generalised anxiety (Johnstone *et al*, 1980; Tyrer *et al*, 1980; Kahn *et al*, 1986; Tyrer *et al*, 1988, 1990). Where treatment effects have been shown, they have applied equally across all diagnoses. If this evidence is accepted it may mean that the diagnostic skills are largely unnecessary once the patient has been regarded as having a neurotic diagnosis of some sort: whatever treatment is chosen would have similar effects across all diagnostic groups.

However, this conclusion has to be qualified. In particular, the phobic disorders have not been satisfactorily included in these comparative studies and, particularly when avoidance behaviour is marked, it is impossible to ignore the importance of behavioural treatment. The same applies to obsessive–compulsive disorder, in which specific behavioural approaches are also successful (Marks *et al*, 1988). In passing, however, it is worth noting that the treatments of phobias and obsessive–compulsive disorders are remarkably similar and certainly the case for distinguishing them could not be made on grounds of treatment alone.

The problem of overlap and co-occurrence of neurotic symptoms has already been discussed, as has the reluctance of classifiers to return to a mixed anxiety/depression diagnostic group (which it is important to note was the accepted classification in the first 40 years of this century). One of the arguments for including a mixed anxiety/depression category is that response to treatment in mixed syndromes is much less satisfactory than when only one mood disturbance is major (Van Valkenburg *et al*, 1984; Stavrakaki & Vargo, 1986; Seivewright & Tyrer, 1990). This is illustrated by the response to treatment in the recent Nottingham study of neurotic disorders (Fig. 10.2). Dysthymic disorder showed a significantly inferior response to treatment than panic and generalised anxiety disorder, and therefore it appears at first sight that depression differs from anxiety in outcome. However, we need to be reminded that dysthymia is a condition which by definition is a chronic one (American Psychiatric Association, 1980) and that in practice it is a mixed diagnosis in which generalised anxiety is an extremely common accompaniment (see Fig. 10.1). Thus the worse response in dysthymia reflects the general finding that mixed anxiety/depression shows a poor response to treatment.

Conclusions

It is much easier to criticise any new solution to an old problem than to provide a constructive alternative. Nevertheless, while the new classifications and atheoretical concepts of neurotic and personality disorders have the

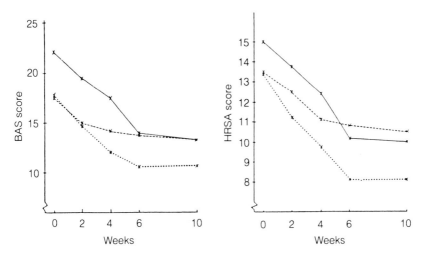

Fig. 10.2. Mean observer (Brief Anxiety Scale; BAS) and self-rated (Hamilton Rating Scale for Anxiety; HRSA) anxiety scores in 73 patients with panic disorder (x———x), 63 with dysthymic disorder (x--------x), and 65 with generalised anxiety disorder (x.........x) (from Tyrer et al (1988), reproduced by permission of the Editor of the Lancet)

appeal of simple measurement and easy understanding, they fail dismally to help clinicians in their daily work. They have been tremendous fillips to the research scientist and to the pharmaceutical industry but are of little value in ordinary practice. They fail primarily because they split diagnosis into compartments that do not accord with clinical reality and only keep them insulated from merger with others by setting arbitrary rules that make no clinical sense. In seeking to be atheoretical, they make the exercise of diagnosis sterile, and while the global explanations of neurosis stemming from psychoanalytical writings are unsatisfactory, one longs for some explanation that goes beyond the mere description of symptoms or behaviour.

Such explanations need to account for a heritable component to both neurosis and personality disorder, the concept of a personality diathesis or vulnerability to neurotic disorder, and the diagnostic change that follows from different life experiences. Some attempts to bring these together are argued for in this account and are summarised in Fig. 10.3. This emphasises the close relationship between personality status and the symptoms of anxiety and depression in the concept of neurotic disorder. Little useful separation of diagnoses can be made until persistent behaviour secondary to mood alters the presentation of the problem: avoidance leading to phobias, ruminations and rituals to obsessive–compulsive disorders, illness behaviour to somatoform disorders, and focus on diet to eating disorders. The combination of anxiety and depression in a single general neurotic syndrome may not be acceptable to those who are bent on splitting diagnosis into ever

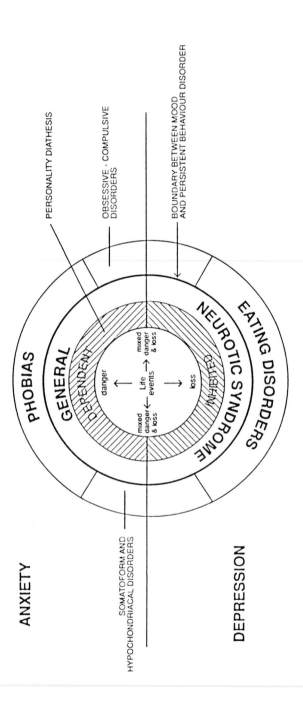

Fig. 10.3. Graphical summary of a single neurotic syndrome

smaller groups, but the pressure for rationalisation will remain while clinicians and patients continue to find the current classification arid, unhelpful and wrong.

References

AMERICAN PSYCHIATRIC ASSOCIATION (1980) *Diagnostic and Statistical Manual of Mental Disorders* (3rd edn) (DSM–III). Washington, DC: APA.
—— (1987) *Diagnostic and Statistical Manual of Mental Disorders* (3rd edn, revised) (DSM–III–R). Washington, DC: APA.
ANDREWS, G., STEWART, G., MORRIS-YATES, A., *et al* (1990) Evidence for a general neurotic syndrome. *British Journal of Psychiatry*, **157**, 6–12.
BAYER, R. & SPITZER, R. L. (1985) Neurosis, psychodynamics and DSM–III: a history of the controversy. *Archives of General Psychiatry*, **42**, 187–196.
BLASHFIELD, R., SPROCK, J., PINKSTON, K., *et al* (1985) Exemplar prototypes of personality disorder diagnoses. *Comprehensive Psychiatry*, **26**, 11–21.
BOYD, J. H., BURKE, J. D., GRUENBERG, E., *et al* (1984) Exclusion criteria of DSM–III: a study of co-occurrence of hierarchy-free syndromes. *Archives of General Psychiatry*, **41**, 983–989.
CASEY, P. R., TYRER, P. J. & PLATT, S. (1985) The relationship between social functioning and psychiatric symptomatology in primary care. *Social Psychiatry*, **20**, 5–9.
DEPARTMENT OF HEALTH AND SOCIAL SECURITY (1989) *Mental Health Statistics for England 1987.* London: Government Statistical Service.
FINLAY-JONES, R. & BROWN, G. W. (1981) Types of stressful life events and the onset of anxiety and depressive disorders. *Psychological Medicine*, **11**, 803–815.
JOHNSTONE, E. C., CUNNINGHAM OWENS, D. G., FRITH, C. D., *et al* (1980) Neurotic illness and its response to anxiolytic and anti-depressant treatment. *Psychological Medicine*, **10**, 321–328.
KAHN, R. J., McNAIR, D. M., LIPMAN, R. S., *et al* (1986) Imipramine and chlordiazepoxide in depressive and anxiety disorders: II. Efficacy in anxious out-patients. *Archives of General Psychiatry*, **43**, 79–85.
KENDELL, R. E. (1976) The classification of depressions: a review of contemporary confusion. *British Journal of Psychiatry*, **129**, 15–28.
KERNBERG, O. F. (1975) *Borderline Conditions and Pathological Narcissism.* New York: Jason Aronson.
KLEIN, D. F. (1964) Delineation of two drug-responsive anxiety syndromes. *Psychopharmacologia*, **5**, 397–408.
—— (1981) Anxiety reconceptualized. In *Anxiety: New Research and Changing Concepts* (eds D. F. Klein & J. G. Rabkin), pp. 235–263. New York: Raven Press.
KOHUT, H. (1971) *The Analysis of the Self.* New York: International Universities Press.
LAZARE, A., KLERMAN, G. L. & ARMOR, D. (1976) Oral, obsessive and hysterical personality patterns. *Archives of General Psychiatry*, **14**, 624–630.
LIEBOWITZ, M. R., FYER, A. J., GORMAN, J. M., *et al* (1988) Tricyclic therapy of the DSM–III anxiety disorders: a review with implications for further research. *Journal of Psychiatric Research*, **22** (suppl. 1), 7–31.
LIVESLEY, W. & JACKSON, D. (1986) The internal consistency and factorial structures of behaviors judged to be associated with DSM–III personality disorders. *American Journal of Psychiatry*, **139**, 1360–1361.
McGLASHAN, T. H. (1983) The borderline syndrome: ii. Is borderline a variant of schizophrenia or affective disorder? *Archives of General Psychiatry*, **40**, 1319–1323.
MARKS, I. M., LELLIOTT, P. T., BASOGLU, M., *et al* (1988) Clomipramine, self-exposure and therapist-aided exposure for obsessive–compulsive rituals. *British Journal of Psychiatry*, **152**, 522–534.

MEDICAL RESEARCH COUNCIL (1965) Report of the Clinical Psychiatry Committee. Clinical trial of the treatment of depressive illness. *British Medical Journal*, i, 881–886.

MONTGOMERY, S. A. (1990) Time for a new approach? Antidepressants as anxiolytics. In *The Anxiolytic Jungle: Where Next?* (ed. D. Wheatley), pp. 128–135. Chichester: Wiley.

POPE, H. G., JONAS, J. M., HUDSON, J. I., et al (1983) The validity of DSM–III borderline personality disorder: a phenomenologic, family history, treatment response and long-term follow-up study. *Archives of General Psychiatry*, **40**, 23–30.

ROBINS, L., HELZER, J., CROUGHAN, J., et al (1979) *The National Institute of Mental Health Diagnostic Interview Schedule*. Rockville: National Institute of Mental Health.

SEIVEWRIGHT, N. & TYRER, P. (1990) Relationship of dysthymia to anxiety and other neurotic disorders. In *Dysthymic Disorder* (eds S. Burton & H. S. Akiskal), pp. 24–36. London: Gaskell.

SLAVNEY, P. R. (1990) *Perspectives on "Hysteria"*. Baltimore: The Johns Hopkins University Press.

SOLOFF, P. H., GEORGE, A., NATHAN, R. S., et al (1986) Progress in pharmacotherapy of borderline disorders: a double blind study of amitriptyline, haloperidol and placebo. *Archives of General Psychiatry*, **43**, 691–697.

SPITZER, R. L. & WILLIAMS, J. B. W. (1983) *Structured Clinical Interview for DSM–III (SCID)*. New York: New York State Psychiatric Institute.

STAVRAKAKI, C. & VARGO, B. (1986) The relationship of anxiety and depression: a review of the literature. *British Journal of Psychiatry*, **149**, 7–16.

TYRER, P. (1985) Neurosis divisible? *Lancet*, i, 685–688.

—— (1989) *Classification of Neurosis*. Chichester: John Wiley.

——, GARDNER, M., LAMBOURN, J., et al (1980) Clinical and pharmacokinetic factors affecting response to phenelzine. *British Journal of Psychiatry*, **136**, 359–365.

——, CASEY, P. & GALL, J. (1983) The relationship between neurosis and personality disorder. *British Journal of Psychiatry*, **142**, 404–408.

——, —— & SEIVEWRIGHT, N. (1986) Common personality features in neurotic disorder. *British Journal of Medical Psychology*, **59**, 289–294.

——, ALEXANDER, J., REMINGTON, M., et al (1987) Relationship between neurotic symptoms and neurotic diagnosis: a longitudinal study. *Journal of Affective Disorders*, **13**, 13–21.

——, SEIVEWRIGHT, N., MURPHY, S., et al (1988) The Nottingham study of neurotic disorder: comparison of drug and psychological treatments. *Lancet*, ii, 235–240.

——, ——, FERGUSON, B., et al (1990) The Nottingham study of neurotic disorder: relationship between personality status and symptoms. *Psychological Medicine*, **20**, 423–431.

UHLENHUTH, E. H., BALTER, M. B., MELLINGER, G. D., et al (1983) Symptom checklist syndromes in the general population: correlations with psychotherapeutic drug use. *Archives of General Psychiatry*, **40**, 1167–1173.

VAN VALKENBURG, C., AKISKAL, H. S., PUZANTIAN, V., et al (1984) Anxious depressions: clinical, family history, and naturalistic outcome – comparisons with panic and major depressive disorders. *Journal of Affective Disorders*, **6**, 67–82.

WIDIGER, T. A. & RODGERS, J. H. (1989) Prevalence and comorbidity of personality disorders. *Psychiatry Annals*, **19**, 786–795.

WORLD HEALTH ORGANIZATION (1988) *International Classification of Diseases*, draft of 10th revision. Geneva: WHO.

11 Nosology and neurosis

PHILIP SNAITH

In company with all medically trained physicians, psychiatrists abhor the absence of a diagnosis. The struggle to arrive at the diagnosis often absorbs more professional effort than the devising and conduct of a successful treatment regime. Whole industries of research effort are devoted to classifying and reclassifying categories of psychiatric disorders, and revisions of revisions of systems are published. The disorders appear in neat lists on the printed page and this procedure provides a general sense of professional security, a structuring of uncertainty and chaos. This comfort lasts only until it is realised that all these categories may coexist, that in fact they are not separate from each other – a phenomenon for which the jargon 'comorbidity' has been introduced.

With the advent of some effective treatments, mainly of the physical variety, diagnostic argument was supported by the observation that some patterns of disorder appeared to respond preferentially to certain treatments. Circular arguments then arose: following the observation that a drug was effective for a certain pattern of disorder, the drug was styled as specific for that disorder and any other condition which also responded to that drug was declared to be an 'atypical' form of the disorder; until, that is, it was finally announced that the treatment, be it electroconvulsive therapy (ECT) or behaviour therapy or some other procedure, was not specific to the disorder that, for instance, ECT was effective in other states than the depressive phase of manic–depressive psychosis and 'behaviour' therapy was not specific to behaviour but altered attitudes and sometimes mood.

In no clinical arena is this more clearly illustrated than in the field of 'depression' and the 'antidepressant' drugs. The first published observation that a drug styled as antidepressant was effective in a disorder dominated by anxiety led to the conclusion that the form of anxiety state was 'atypical depression' (West & Dally, 1959). The later observation that a similar disorder responded to another antidepressant drug led to the conclusion not that the disorder was a form of depression, but that it had special clinical features which justified its dissociation from the body of anxiety disorders. Thus 'panic disorder' was conceived and ICD–10 (World Health Organization, 1987) follows DSM–III–R (American Psychiatric Association, 1987) in the recognition of a separate category with peculiar affiliations, that is, panic disorder (with agoraphobia), panic disorder (without agoraphobia) and agoraphobia (with or without a history of panic disorder). Commenting upon this famous observation Klein (1981) wrote:

> "Our early observations on imipramine were received like the proverbial lead balloon because of the general conviction that antidepressants should not affect anxiety and that it was ridiculous to think a drug might selectively benefit severe anxiety more than mild anxiety. Of course the simplest hypothesis was that I was misdiagnosing depression as William Sargant pointed out to me in a personal communication."

The observation that 'antidepressant' drugs are effective in some forms of severe anxiety state, including those in which there are sudden fit-like episodes of overwhelming anxiety with autonomic manifestations, is now overwhelming (Modigh, 1987; Liebowitz, 1989) but there has been staunch rearguard reaction to the observation and entrenched defence of the position that anxiety states are 'neurotic' and must therefore be treated by psychotherapeutic means. Indeed when, as a novice in the field of psychiatry, I presented a case as one of endogenous anxiety and considered antidepressant treatment, I was firmly advised to consider practice in some other branch of medicine. The fact is now of course dawning that the so-called 'antidepressant' drugs have a wider range of therapeutic action than in the field of the depressive disorders (Murphy *et al*, 1985).

Classification of psychiatric disorders is not a useless exercise; some sort of ordering is necessary. It is necessary for the making of proper returns to administrative departments of patients admitted to psychiatric hospitals and it helps authors of texts to arrange their material and their students to read it. But too close an adherence to the categories provided by systems of classification carries danger for both research and clinical management. Hysteria is a prototype of all neurotic disorder and certainly the one which Sigmund Freud could most confidently pronounce to be a 'psychoneurosis'. Hysteria, as we shall see, has now gone but the ghost of the 'tough old word' lingers to haunt us and to provide salutary warning: the diagnosis of hysteria, said Eliot Slater, is not only a snare but a delusion (Slater, 1965).

Depressive disorders

The term 'neurotic' in association with 'depression' is likely to linger in psychiatric parlance for longer than in any other clinical context. The introduction of 'dysthymia' has not so far found wide acceptance. Dysthymia is defined in terms of a relatively mild but persisting disorder of mood; DSM–III–R requires that there should be a two-year period in which the person is never without depressive symptoms for more than two months; this implies that the disorder may be manifest as brief recurrent depressive episodes. The depressive symptoms listed in the definition of dysthymia are: poor appetite *or* overeating, insomnia *or* hypersomnia, low energy or fatigue, low self-esteem, poor concentration or difficulty making decisions, and feelings of hopelessness. The two major manifestations of the DSM–III–R category of major depressive episode, depressed mood and anhedonia, are not included in the list of dysthymic symptoms; nor, it may be noted, is anxiety included. True to the atheoretical nature of DSM–III–R, no suggestion is given as to the aetiology of the disorder apart from the fact that it may not be secondary to other psychiatric and physical disorders. ICD–9 (World Health Organization, 1978), on the other hand, defined the state of neurotic depression as having *usually* ensued after a distressing experience and that there is *often* a preoccupation with the psychic trauma which preceded the disorder. The revision, ICD–10, also proposes to abolish the concept of depressive neurosis and indeed to banish mild depressive and dysthymic states from the company of neurotic disorder. The concept of a depressive state consequent upon stress is henceforth to be called an 'adjustment disorder'.

More confusion has surrounded the term 'depression' than any other concept in psychiatry and yet depressive disorders occupy more time of most psychiatrists than any other disorder. The term 'depression' was introduced as a replacement for 'melancholia'. It was the confident opinion of Adolf Meyer (1905) that the adoption of the term would lead to clarification. Yet this was not to be the case, either in the sense of a disorder or a symptom, where it is generally used for a poorly defined state of misery or, as in the case of the definition used in the Present State Examination (Wing *et al*, 1974), for a mixture of concepts. In a comment on the status of neurotic depression, Ascher (1952) wrote:

> "There appears to be a good deal of confusion . . . about depressive illness which is a left-over from the era of descriptive psychiatry. Concepts of psychogenesis, endogeny, reactivity, neurosis, psychosis have been introduced to clarify the issue . . . without producing the desired result."

There was no problem with the recognition of a *severe* depressive state which might alternate with manic episodes and which was considered to be a form of psychosis, but all disorders which exist in severe form may also occur in milder forms and the *mild* form of the psychotic or endogenous depression was never defined nor guidance given for its recognition (Snaith, 1987). It shaded imperceptibly into neurotic depression, and Kendell (1976) was to comment that severity was the only distinguishing factor between 'psychotic' and 'neurotic' forms of depressive disorder. Since anxiety, obsessions, irritability, and other neurotic symptoms occur in both severe and milder forms of depressive disorder there was still greater difficulty in distinguishing between depressive neurosis and the mild form of the psychotic depressive state. Akiskal *et al* (1978) listed the characteristics which are usually ascribed to the concept of neurotic depression:

(a) preservation of reality testing, i.e. lack of delusional ideation and preservation of insight
(b) mildness of the disorder
(c) coexistence of 'neurotic' symptoms of obsessions, anxiety, phobias and depersonalisation
(d) psychogenesis, i.e. the disorder is caused by stressful circumstances, especially loss of events
(e) there is an underlying vulnerable personality structure predisposing to the disorder.

There are however no characteristic symptoms distinguishing between neurotic, stress-related depressive disorder and the mild forms of the psychotic disorder unless they be the 'biological' symptoms of weight loss, early-morning waking, and diurnal variation. These are unreliable symptoms – diurnal variation is frequently absent or reversed, weight loss may depend on the duration of the illness and be caused by concurrent somatic disease, and insomnia is determined by a number of factors including age, old people tending naturally to wake earlier.

Klein (1974) proposed that a distinction could be made on the basis of other symptoms and considered that the pathognomonic feature of the mild biogenic (endogenous) depressive state is "A sharp, unreactive, pervasive impairment of the capacity to experience pleasure or to respond affectively to the anticipation of pleasure". This is the state of anhedonia, an experience which is quite distinct and may be differentiated from the concept of depressed mood which is more difficult to define precisely and occurs in the wide variety of expressions of unhappiness, misery, demoralisation or pessimism.

The DSM in its previous edition (DSM–III; American Psychiatric Association, 1980) considered that a disorder to be called major depression could be defined on the presence of ten symptoms, one of which must be dysphoric (depressed) mood and another anhedonia, defined as "loss of interest in all or almost all usual activities and pastimes"; only one of these two symptoms need be present to qualify for the diagnosis and there must in addition be another four symptoms from a list of eight; the revised (DSM–III–R) requirements for the diagnosis of major depressive episode are similar.

An interesting change between the two versions of the DSM is with regard to the new category of dysthymia. Whereas the former version required the presence of much the same list of symptoms as in the category of major depressive episode although "not of sufficient severity and duration to meet the criteria of Major Depressive Episode", the revision excludes the symptoms indicating a severe disorder: psychomotor retardation or agitation and recurrent suicidal ideation or attempt at suicide. The symptom of anhedonia is *also* excluded, which seems to indicate recognition that it has some special significance and that, if present, the diagnosis of major depressive disorder should be made.

The revisers of the ICD have also recognised the special significance of anhedonia; the concept of 'somatic' depression (probably equivalent to endogenous or biogenic depression) has been put forward, defined in terms of the presence of the 'biological' symptoms – weight loss, early waking, diurnal variation and, in addition, psychomotor retardation, agitation and anhedonia with lack of response of mood to circumstances (lack of reactivity). Anhedonia seems to be increasingly recognised as a distinguishing feature between endogenous (somatic, biogenic) depressive disorder and the form of depressive disorder which has been called depressive neurosis or dysthymia.

When we were asked in the early 1980s to design a simple self-assessment scale to assist in the detection of a disorder which might benefit from the prescription of antidepressant drugs, we devised the Hospital Anxiety and Depression (HAD) scale (Zigmond & Snaith, 1983) which separated the concepts of anxiety and depression, and avoided items likely to be unduly influenced by the presence of somatic disorder. It had a major component (five of the seven depression subscale items) of anhedonia.

The situation regarding the recognition of different forms of depressive disorder remains confused; indeed one commentator (van Praag, 1990) wrote:

> "The proposed dichotomy (major depression and dysthymia) resembles two poorly focussed slides projected simultaneously and largely overlapping. Clarity is far to seek. The state of affairs is detrimental to research as well as for clinical practice. In biological psychiatry the search is for biological underpinnings of specific syndromes. . . . These goals are ill served by diagnostic ambiguities."

It is certain that more thought and research needs to be given to this important topic if available treatments are to be rationally and effectively used. There is nothing more futile than the prescription of potentially toxic antidepressant drugs to unhappy people who cannot be expected to respond to such medication; conversely there is no greater waste of the resources of limited psychotherapeutic time and expensive expertise than prolonged treatment in an attempt to relieve depressive disorders which would have responded to a few weeks of judicious prescribing of an antidepressant drug.

Apart from those special forms of anxiety state which require pharmaco-therapy, anxiety states and phobic disorders generally respond to one of the varieties of psychotherapeutic anxiety management techniques. The danger of prescribing, and subsequently blindly following, a treatment procedure according to the initial diagnosis of the case is underlined in this field by the fact that the anxiety state frequently commences in the setting of a biogenic depressive disorder which may then subside but re-emerge at a later stage, possibly after treatment has commenced, and effectively block further progress with the psychotherapeutic procedure. Figure 11.1 illustrates this as charted by the HAD scores; treatment of the emerging depressive disorder enabled the anxiety management procedure to continue to a satisfactory conclusion.

Obsessional disorders

The phenomena of the obsessional disorders provide a source of clinical fascination; the symbolism is intriguing and perplexing but in many cases, as in the washing and checking rituals, there appears to be a distortion of a search for security, a fending off of potential disaster but with ludicrous progression to time-wasting behaviour over which the individual has lost

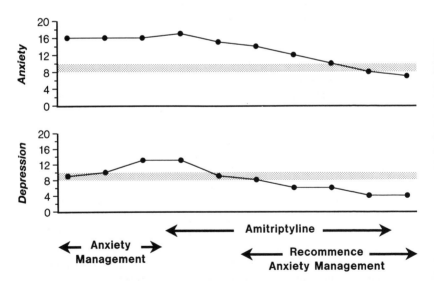

Fig. 11.1. *The management of a single patient originally presenting with an anxiety disorder is illustrated by charting the scores over time on the anxiety and depression subscales of the HAD. The shaded region indicates the cut-off mark for 'cases' (from Snaith, 1991, by permission of the Oxford University Press). (For information concerning the supply of the HAD scale and chart, send an addressed envelope to the author)*

control. Other forms of mental activity included under the rubric of obsessive–compulsive phenomena include the endless chains of thought, often upon metaphysical and unanswerable themes, or the counting of objects or performance of meaningless arithmetical computations. Other such phenomena include the appearance before the mind's eye of mental imagery often of an alarming sexual or aggressive nature. There may be fear-laden thoughts of losing control and committing some atrocious act of self-harm or harm to others; the feared act may be less disastrous but would still lead to extreme social embarrassment or disgrace were it to occur and frequently the theme is that of making obscene sounds or gestures in a public place, especially one where prudery or piety normally prevails.

The cumbersome hybrid term 'obsessive–compulsive' betrays a certain attempt to assemble, under the rubric of a single category, groups of phenomena which are not certainly related either by regular syndromal co-occurrence or by some common pathogenic mechanism. The term 'obsession' would imply a constant preoccupation with a particular theme and 'compulsion' implies a driven form of behaviour overwhelming any possible will to resist engaging in it. There have been many attempts at definition of the core features of a disorder to be categorised as obsessive–compulsive. The major elements which have been isolated are those of: (a) a sense of compulsion to engage in the act or thought, (b) a resistance or attempt not to be so engaged, (c) a recognition of the senselessness of the activity, and (d) an admission of the thought leading to the activity being one's own and not imposed by others – in Lewis's words (1936) "home-made but disowned" or, in the modern jargon, 'ego-dystonic'. There is also a frequent pervasive sensation of 'something left unfinished', which Pierre Janet (1907) called the "*sentiments d'incomplétude*". Not all these features are present in every case and there has been endless argument as to whether any of them should be considered to be a necessary feature for a disorder to be stated to be 'obsessive–compulsive'. ICD-10 proposes that the second part of the term should be dropped and the disorder, and its phenomena, referred to more simply and euphoniously by the first term alone (i.e. obsessional acts, obsessional thoughts and so on).

The attempt to force this assemblage of phenomena into a single category, with implication of common pathogenic mechanisms and common response to treatment, is not successful. Moreover it seems to imply that some basic similarity in the treatment approaches should prevail and therapeutic response should be similar. This is manifestly not the case. The psychodynamic explanations, commencing with Freud's own attempt to unravel the complex disorders, have never been successful; they defy understanding in such terms and despite his heroic attempt to construct a theory based upon reaction formation to aggressive impulses unresolved at the 'anal' stage of development, he had to admit: "It must be confessed that, if we endeavour to penetrate more deeply into its nature [of the obsessional neurosis] we still have to rely upon doubtful assumptions and unconfirmed suspicions'' (Freud, 1926).

The behaviourist explanations, naive in their conception, started off with no such doubts: the phenomena of obsessional disorders were to be considered as anxiety-relieving devices and their very success in relief of anxiety leads to their perpetuation. Unfortunately for such a neat theory it was the observations of clinicians (Walker & Beech, 1969) that carrying out the obsessional rituals did *not* relieve anxiety and indeed some patients became *more* anxious as they continued the behaviour. Other theorists, including those espousing the so-called 'cognitive' view, have had no greater success in providing an explanation or a successful method of treatment. One method did find wide acclaim and that was based upon the prevention of engagement in the behaviour (so-called 'response prevention') but the studies which seemed to confirm the success of the method were flawed by the combined use of antidepressant drugs with the behavioural treatment.

Many disorders are characterised by abnormal behaviour which the subject recognises as senseless, embarrassing and harmful, behaviour which is both ego-dystonic and yet carried out under irresistible compulsion. Examples are some cases of exhibitionism (Snaith, 1983), trichotillomania and bulimia nervosa. Although these conditions are characterised by a sense of compulsion they are not usually considered to be obsessional disorders. The most interesting development in the approach to understanding the enigma of obsessional phenomena comes from the observation of their link with organic brain disorders and to disorders which, by reason of reliable response to antidepressant and other psychotic drugs, may be considered to be based upon disordered function of neurotransmitter systems. The older observation that obsessional symptoms occur in post-encephalitic Parkinsonism has recently been supported by an association of obsessions with the aftermath of Sydenham's chorea. Perhaps the most intriguing observation is the association of the Tourette's syndrome with obsessional phenomena (Pauls *et al*, 1986; Robertson, 1989; Trimble, 1989). There is now an emphasis on the analysis of the association between obsessional disorders and basal ganglia dysfunction (Stahl, 1988; Rapoport, 1990). Evidence of abnormal functioning of the basal ganglia and frontal cortex in obsessional disorder is now emerging from positron emission tomography (PET) studies (Bench *et al*, 1990). There is also emphasis on the observation that certain 'antidepressant' drugs, those acting preferentially on the serotonergic neurotransmitter system, are especially effective in the treatment of obsessional disorders.

In DSM–III–R obsessive–compulsive disorders are categorised with the anxiety disorders. Perhaps it does not matter too much which of the categories of disorders receives these elusive states; what matters is a recognition of the features that may lead to successful intervention. Certainly the observations that have led the compilers of ICD–10 to stress the frequent association with mood disorder places an emphasis upon the only treatment intervention, short of psychosurgery, that has been reliably shown to lead to relief of some obsessional disorders – antidepressant drugs (Zohar & Insel, 1987).

Somatoform and dissociative disorders

Hysteria, the archetype of all neurotic disorders, is a concept that has undergone many transmutations. The term has stood service for a great variety of concepts since it was first proposed that the uterus might take leave of its moorings in the pelvis and cause symptoms in many parts of the body. This ancient idea was probably based upon an astute clinical observation that the turbulent emotion and multiple symptoms associated with disorder of the temporal lobe of the brain are associated with a characteristic sensation of swelling arising from the pelvis and passing upward through the body. This sensation was the origin of the term 'globus hystericus' which is now, inappropriately, applied to a sensation of a lump in the throat causing difficulty in swallowing. In the course of time a great many concepts were merged and 'hysteria' became a ragbag of "multiple manifestations of semantic confusion" (Cleghorn, 1969). The major concepts were those of suggestibility, gain, distorted communication, multiple symptoms, dramatisation and a variable constellation of personality characteristics which Chodoff & Lyons (1958) summed up as: "A picture of women in the words of men, a caricature of femininity". In addition to all this it became a term of opprobrium, signifying an exasperation of the clinician with the patient:

> "It appears on the case sheet most readily if the doctor has found himself at a loss, if the case is obscure or if the treatment has been unsuccessful. Of all diagnoses it is that which is least likely to have been made in a spirit of detachment." (Slater & Glithero, 1965)

Freud's view of hysteria, which came to dominate psychiatric formulations, as a disorder with prominent somatisation leading to loss of function, followed the publication of his thoughts, with Breuer, of the case of 'Anna O'. The appearance of the functional loss appeared to fit neatly with the observation of serene unconcern, or *belle indifférence*, about the disability and the assumption was drawn that emotional suffering from psychic trauma had been made less distressing by the psychic defence of 'conversion' of the affect into the physical symptom. This view gained wide credence, but the supposed lack of concern about the disability was not always present and emotional distress in the form of prominent anxiety and depression frequently persisted. The views of Janet regarding hysteria, or at least some aspects of that bewildering group of disorders, were eclipsed by Freud (Nemiah, 1989). Janet (1907), in his *The Major Symptoms of Hysteria*, had focused attention on the concept of *désagrégation* which was translated into English as 'dissociation'. His view of loss of integration of some aspect of personal (psychic or somatic) function with the normally integrated functions of memory, identity and consciousness, was based upon a view of some underlying psychic weakness:

> "Hysteria is a malady of personal synthesis . . . a form of mental depression characterised by a tendency to dissociation and emancipation of the systems of ideas and functions which constitute personality. . . . The starting point of hysteria is the same as that of most great neuroses, it is a depression, an exhaustion of the higher centres of the encephalon."

Although Janet did not deny the importance of psychic trauma in the genesis of hysteria, he proposed that there was a sort of *physioneurosis* to be set against Freud's confident proclamation of a *psychoneurosis*. The observation of the 'serene unconcern' about a disability or loss of function was more simply explained than in the Freudian hypothesis: one cannot be concerned about something of which one is not aware.

There is certainly no clear separation of the symptom patterns commonly called hysteria from the states of anxiety and other emotional turmoil. Frequently classic symptoms, such as loss of personal identity with wandering (fugue state), are seen in the setting of depressive illness, and Stengel (1941, 1943) proposed that the fugue was a form of 'suicidal equivalent' in a depressed person. Likewise, Kennedy & Neville (1957) considered that psychogenic amnesia may occur in the setting of the aftermath of head injury; indeed organic disease of the central nervous system is particularly likely to provoke the 'hysterical elaboration' of greater disability (Whitlock, 1967; Slater & Roth, 1969; Merskey & Buhrich, 1975), a view more in keeping with Janet's observations than with Freudian theory.

The demise of the term 'hysteria' in the present revision of classifications of disorders is to be welcomed. The concept of dissociative disorders is now introduced in both the ICD and the DSM systems; these are to be considered alongside somatoform disorders. DSM–III–R, but not ICD–10, provides a separate category for conversion disorder. The attempt to create separate diagnostic categories for states of distress presenting with prominent somatic symptoms has led to the term 'somatisation disorder' and, where pain is the major symptom, 'somatoform pain disorder'. Somatisation disorder owes its existence to the powerful lobby and multiple publications from a group in the USA who promoted the French physician Dr Briquet to eponymous fame. In order to qualify for the diagnosis of Briquet's syndrome a person must have had a complicated medical history commencing before the age of 35, to have suffered at various times from at least 25 symptoms selected from nine out of ten groups of symptoms, to have no other diagnosis to explain the symptoms and, true to old stereotypes concerning hysteria, to be female. How males were to be classified was never made quite clear; perhaps the diagnostician always stopped counting symptoms before he reached the critical number of 25. The fallacies associated with this diagnosis have been outlined (Snaith, 1968*a,b*; *Lancet*, 1977).

Pain occupies a special position as a symptom eliciting a caring response and there are separate categories of somatoform pain disorder (DSM–III–R) and persistent pain disorder (ICD–10). The definitions in both systems recognise that emotional factors *may* play a part in the causation of the disorder but both definitions are unsatisfactory; if there are emotional factors and personal problems as the basis of the pain it is surely better to focus attention upon them than to mask the basic problem by a spurious categorical label. States of anxiety and depression are often the basis of somatisation and treatment of the emotional disorder will often lead to resolution of the somatic symptoms. The creation of diagnostic categories carries the risk of labelling and ignoring of the underlying condition.

In DSM–III–R, two concepts are included in the definition of hypo-chondriacal disorder: a fear of disease and a conviction of the presence of disease despite informed assurance to the contrary. Many factors contribute to the perception of bodily sensations and their transmutation to persisting distress requiring medical attention (Mayou, 1976; Mechanic, 1986). The attempt to forge a unitary category of hypochondriacal disorder is unhelpful and would not have been necessary if the classification systems had made provision for fear, or phobia, of illness along with other phobias.

Conclusions

The patterns of disorder which traditionally are called 'neuroses' were once considered to be due to an abnormality of neural function. Under the influence of Freud the term 'psychoneurosis' came into wider use; this implies that the disorders must be understood in terms of stress, characteristic patterns of reaction, or 'defence mechanisms' to limit the suffering caused by the stress, and a vulnerable personality structure which was also formed under the same influences. Older observations were forgotten or suppressed and the possibility of some form of constitutional predisposition was put on one side. The potentially productive ideas of Pierre Janet were submerged under the flood of the new psychoanalytic teaching stemming from Freud and his followers (Nemiah, 1989). These ideas are being rediscovered together with the revival of interest in the biological basis of some aspects of neurotic disorder. The simple categorisation of patterns of disorder into diagnostic compartments is no longer justified. In Chapter 10 Tyrer has reviewed the evidence, including the conclusions from his own studies, that patterns of disorder do not remain fixed but change in a kaleidoscopic manner throughout the course of the person's life.

The changing patterns are not confined to the disorders called neuroses but occur also in the other great category, the psychoses. Moreover 'neurotic' and 'psychotic' patterns are frequently mixed. Sometimes psychotic disorders are preceded by neurotic symptoms and sometimes, after the more florid symptoms have subsided, the residual disability appears to be 'neurotic' rather than 'psychotic' (Cheadle *et al*, 1978; *British Medical Journal*, 1978). Depressive illness is frequently preceded by anxiety symptoms (Walker, 1959); anxiety and other neurotic symptoms, such as obsessions, frequently persist after recovery from the affective psychosis in the manner that Janet so well described. Today the emphasis on a 'new' category of anxiety state, so-called panic disorder, has been examined from many points of view and the links with depressive illness are confirmed (Stavrakaki & Vargo, 1986; Breier *et al*, 1985).

In the area of obsessional symptoms the borderline between 'neurotic' and 'psychotic' forms of the disorders has always been a source of fascination for psychopathologists (Lewis, 1936; Insel & Akiskal, 1986).

Great effort is devoted to the construction of diagnostic classification. Psychiatrists are encouraged to believe that once the diagnosis is made, the correct treatment will follow. Unfortunately treatment is prescribed by diagnostic category rather than by the needs of the patient at that point in the course of the disorder.

In a survey of the nosological status of schizophrenia Hays (1984) came to the conclusion that psychiatrists were blinkered by their diagnostic categories. If this may be the case in the area of psychotic disorder it is even more true for the changing patterns called 'neurotic disorders'.

References

AMERICAN PSYCHIATRIC ASSOCIATION (1980) *Diagnostic and Statistical Manual of Mental Disorders* (3rd edn) (DSM–III). Washington, DC: APA.
—— (1987) *Diagnostic and Statistical Manual of Mental Disorders* (3rd edn, revised) (DSM–III–R). Washington, DC: APA.
AKISKAL, H. S., BITAR, A. H., PUZANTIAN, V. R., *et al* (1978) The nosological status of neurotic depression. *Archives of General Psychiatry*, **35**, 756–766.
ASCHER, F. (1952) A criticism of the concept of neurotic depression. *American Journal of Psychiatry*, **108**, 901–908.
BENCH, C. J., DOLAN, R. J., FRISTON, K. J., *et al* (1990) Positron emission tomography in the study of brain metabolism in psychiatric and neuropsychiatric disorders. *British Journal of Psychiatry*, **157** (suppl. 9), 82–95.
BREIER, A., CHARNEY, D. & HENINGER, G. R. (1985) The diagnostic validity of anxiety disorders and their relationship to depressive illness. *American Journal of Psychiatry*, **142**, 787–797.
BRITISH MEDICAL JOURNAL (1978) Is schizophrenia a psychosis or a neurosis? *British Medical Journal*, *iii*, 76.

CHEADLE, A. J., FREEMAN, H. L. & KORER, J. (1978) Chronic schizophrenic patients in the community. *British Journal of Psychiatry*, **132**, 221–227.
CHODOFF, P. & LYONS, H. (1958) Hysteria, the hysterical personality and hysterical conversion. *American Journal of Psychiatry*, **114**, 734–740.
CLEGHORN, R. A. (1969) Hysteria – multiple manifestations of semantic confusion. *Canadian Psychiatric Association Journal*, **14**, 539–551.
FREUD, S. (1926) Inhibitions, symptoms and anxiety. In *Standard Edition of the Complete Psychological Works, Vol. 20* (ed. J. Strachey). London: Hogarth Press.
HAYS, P. (1984) The nosological status of schizophrenia. *Lancet*, i, 1342–1344.
INSEL, T. R. & AKISKAL, H. S. (1986) Obsessive–compulsive disorder with psychotic features: a phenomenologic analysis. *American Journal of Psychiatry*, **143**, 1527–1533.
JANET, P. (1907) *The Major Symptoms of Hysteria*. New York: Macmillan.
KENDELL, R. E. (1976) The classification of depression: a review. *British Journal of Psychiatry*, **129**, 15–28.
KENNEDY, A. & NEVILLE, J. (1957) Sudden loss of memory. *British Medical Journal*, ii, 428–433.
KLEIN, D. F. (1974) Endogenomorphic depression. *Archives of General Psychiatry*, **31**, 447–454.
—— (1981) Anxiety reconceptualized. In *Anxiety, New Research and Changing Concepts* (eds D. F. Klein & J. G. Rabkin). New York: Raven Press.
LANCET (1977) Briquet's syndrome or hysteria? *Lancet*, i, 1139.
LEWIS, A. J. (1936) Problems of obsessional illness. *Proceedings of the Royal Society of Medicine*, **29**, 325–326.
LIEBOWITZ, M. R. (1989) Antidepressants in panic disorders. *British Journal of Psychiatry*, **155** (suppl. 6), 46–52.
MAYOU, R. (1976) The nature of bodily symptoms. *British Journal of Psychiatry*, **129**, 55–60.
MECHANIC, D. (1986) The concept of illness behaviour: culture situation and personal disposition. *Psychological Medicine*, **16**, 1–7.
MERSKEY, H. & BUHRICH, N. A. (1975) Hysteria and organic brain disease. *British Journal of Medical Psychology*, **48**, 359–365.
MEYER, A. (1905) Discussant: in the classification of melancholia. *Journal of Nervous Mental Diseases*, **32**, 112–117.
MODIGH, K. (1987) Antidepressant drugs in anxiety disorders. *Acta Psychiatrica Scandinavica*, **76** (suppl. 335), 57–71.
MURPHY, D. L., SIEVER, L. J. & INSEL, T. R. (1985) Therapeutic responses to tricyclic antidepressants and related drugs in non-affective disorder patient populations. *Progress in Neuropsychopharmacology and Biological Psychiatry*, **9**, 3–13.
NEMIAH, J. C. (1989) Janet Redivivus: the centenary of *L'automatisine psychologique. American Journal of Psychiatry*, **146**, 1527–1529.
PAULS, D. L., TOWBIN, K., LECKMAN, J. F., et al (1986) Gilles de la Tourette's syndrome and obsessive–compulsive disorder. *Archives of General Psychiatry*, **43**, 1180–1182.
RAPOPORT, J. L. (1990) Obsessive–compulsive disorder and basal ganglia dysfunction. *Psychological Medicine*, **20**, 465–469.
ROBERTSON, M. M. (1989) The Gilles de la Tourette syndrome: the current status. *British Journal of Psychiatry*, **154**, 147–169.
SLATER, E. (1965) Diagnosis of 'hysteria'. *British Medical Journal*, i, 1395–1399.
—— & GLITHERO, E. (1965) A follow-up study of patients diagnosed as suffering from hysteria. *Journal of Psychosomatic Research*, **9**, 9–13.
—— & ROTH, M. (1969) *Clinical Psychiatry* (3rd edn). London: Ballière.
SNAITH, R. P. (1968a) Concepts of hysteria (letter). *British Journal of Psychiatry*, **114**, 1593–1594.
—— (1968b) Family and marital hysteria (letter). *British Journal of Psychiatry*, **114**, 644–645.
—— (1983) Exhibitionism: a clinical conundrum. *British Journal of Psychiatry*, **143**, 231–235.
—— (1987) The concepts of mild depression. *British Journal of Psychiatry*, **150**, 387–393.
—— (1991) *Clinical Neurosis* (2nd edn). Oxford: Oxford University Press.
STAHL, S. M. (1988) Basal ganglia neuropharmacology and obsessive–compulsive disorder: the obsessive–compulsive disorder hypothesis of basal ganglia dysfunction. *Psychopharmacological Bulletin*, **24**, 370–374.

STAVRAKAKI, C. & VARGO, B. (1986) The relationship of anxiety and depression: a review of the literature. *British Journal of Psychiatry*, **149**, 7–16.

STENGEL, E. (1941) On the aetiology of fugue states. *Journal of Mental Science*, **87**, 572–599.

—— (1943) Further studies of pathological wandering. *Journal of Mental Science*, **89**, 224–241.

TRIMBLE, M. (1989) Psychopathology and movement disorders: a perspective of the Gilles de la Tourette syndrome. *Journal of Neurology, Neurosurgery and Psychiatry* (special supplement), 90–95.

VAN PRAAG, H. M. (1990) The DSM IV (depression) classification: to be or not to be? *Journal of Nervous and Mental Disorders*, **178**, 147–149.

WALKER, L. (1959) The prognosis of affective illness with overt anxiety. *Journal of Neurology, Neurosurgery and Psychiatry*, **22**, 338–341.

WALKER, V. J. & BEECH, J. R. (1969) Mood state and ritualistic behaviour of obsessional patients. *British Journal of Psychiatry*, **115**, 1261–1268.

WEST, E. D. & DALLY, P. J. (1959) The effects of iproniazid in depressive syndromes. *British Medical Journal*, i, 1491–1494.

WHITLOCK, F. A. (1967) The aetiology of hysteria. *Acta Psychiatrica Scandinavica*, **43**, 144–162.

WING, J. K., COOPER, J. E. & SARTORIUS, N. (1974) *The Measurement and Classification of Psychiatric Symptoms*. London: Cambridge University Press.

WORLD HEALTH ORGANIZATION (1978) *Mental Disorders: Glossary and Guide to their Classification in Accordance with the Ninth Revision of the International Classification of Diseases* (ICD-9). Geneva: WHO.

—— (1987) *International Classification of Diseases*, draft of 10th revision. Geneva: WHO.

ZIGMOND, A. & SNAITH, R. P. (1983) The Hospital Anxiety and Depression Scale. *Acta Psychiatrica Scandinavica*, **67**, 361–370.

ZOHAR, J. & INSEL, T. R. (1987) Drug treatment of obsessive–compulsive disorders. *Journal of Affective Disorders*, **13**, 193–202.

Index

Compiled by **STANLEY THORLEY**